FITNESS:
Achieving a Toned and Shaped Body

Contents

Introduction

Physical fitness is a cornerstone of overall wellbeing, encompassing a state of health and the capacity to execute everyday tasks with enthusiasm and attentiveness. Understanding its importance is crucial to adopting a lifestyle that prioritizes both mental and physical health.

Understanding the Importance of Physical Fitness

Physical fitness goes beyond mere aesthetics; it is about cultivating a lifestyle that enhances the quality of life. At its core, physical fitness refers to the body's capacity to perform efficiently and successfully in both professional and recreational endeavors, to fight sickness, and to handle unanticipated demands. This section delves into the multifaceted significance of physical fitness.

Enhanced Cardiovascular Health: Regular exercise strengthens the heart, enabling it to pump blood more efficiently. This, in turn, improves circulation, reduces the risk of heart disease, and maintains optimal blood pressure levels. Understanding the connection between exercise and cardiovascular health is vital for preventing conditions like heart attacks and strokes.

Weight Management: Physical fitness plays a pivotal function in weight control. Regular physical exercise helps burn calories, which aids in weight reduction or maintenance. This is critical for avoiding obesity, which is linked to a variety of health concerns such as diabetes, hypertension, and joint difficulties.

Muscle Strength and Endurance: A fit body is characterized by well-developed muscles that provide strength and endurance. Understanding the importance of muscle strength goes beyond aesthetics; it directly influences daily activities, promoting better posture, balance, and overall functionality. This is particularly significant as we age and face natural declines in muscle mass.

Mental Health Benefits: Physical fitness is intrinsically linked to psychological health. Exercise triggers the production of endorphins, which are naturally occurring chemicals that improve mood. This connection between physical activity and mental health underscores the importance of fitness in managing stress, anxiety, and depression.

Improved Immune System: Regular exercise boosts the immune system, strengthening the body's defenses against illnesses and infections. Understanding how physical activity enhances immune function is crucial, especially in the context of preventing illnesses and promoting overall health.

Enhanced Flexibility and Range of Motion: Physical fitness encompasses flexibility, this is essential for maintaining the joints' whole range of motion. Stretching exercises and activities like yoga contribute to improved flexibility, reducing the risk of injuries, and enhancing overall mobility.

Disease Prevention: A sedentary lifestyle is a significant risk factor for various chronic diseases. Understanding the role of physical fitness in preventing conditions such as diabetes, certain cancers, and osteoporosis emphasizes the proactive approach one can take to safeguard their health through regular exercise.

Boosted energy levels: Contrary to common belief, engaging in physical activity boosts energy levels rather than depleting them. Regular exercise enhances cardiovascular function and improves the efficiency of oxygen and nutrient delivery to tissues, promoting sustained energy throughout the day.

In conclusion, understanding the importance of physical fitness extends beyond the confines of a gym. It is about recognizing the intricate interplay between exercise and overall health, both physical and mental. Embracing a lifestyle that prioritizes physical fitness sets the foundation for a fulfilling and resilient life where individuals can actively participate in the experiences that bring them joy and satisfaction. As we explore various facets of physical fitness, it becomes evident that it is not a luxury but an essential component of a holistic approach to health and wellbeing.

The evolution of fitness gyms is a fascinating journey that mirrors changing attitudes towards health, wellness, and physical exercise. From humble beginnings to the modern, multifaceted establishments we see today, fitness gyms have undergone a remarkable transformation.

The Evolution of Fitness Gyms

Early Beginnings: The concept of communal exercise spaces dates back to ancient civilizations. In Greece, gymnasiums were hubs for physical and intellectual activities, fostering a holistic approach to education. Similarly, in ancient Rome, public baths served as places for exercise and socialization. These early spaces laid the groundwork for the idea that physical well-being is interconnected with mental and social aspects.

Rise of Home Gyms: The early 20th century saw a surge in home-based exercise equipment, fueled by the desire for convenience and privacy. Simple apparatus like dumbbells, barbells, and resistance bands became popular for home use. However, the communal aspect of working out was somewhat lost during this period, as individuals tended to focus on personal fitness within the confines of their homes.

The Fitness Revolution: The 1970s marked a significant turning point with the emergence of the fitness revolution. Influenced by changing societal attitudes towards health and appearance, people began to seek structured workout routines. This era witnessed the birth of commercial fitness centers, catering to the growing demand for specialized equipment and professional guidance. These gyms laid the foundation for the modern fitness industry, introducing concepts like aerobics and group classes.

Introduction to High-Tech Equipment:
As technology advanced, so did the equipment available in fitness gyms. The late 20th century and early 21st century witnessed the integration of high-tech exercise machines, electronic fitness

trackers, and virtual reality-enhanced workouts. This technological evolution not only made workouts more engaging but also allowed for precise monitoring of individual progress.

Focus on specialized training. In recent years, there has been a shift towards specialized training facilities catering to specific fitness niches. Cross Fit boxes, yoga studios, and HIIT (high-intensity interval training) facilities have grown in popularity, providing customized exercises to suit a variety of tastes. This diversity is a reflection of the knowledge that every person has different requirements and objectives and that there is no one-size-fits-all approach to fitness.

Incorporation of Wellness Services: Modern fitness gyms have evolved beyond being just places to lift weights or run on treadmills. Many now offer a holistic approach to wellbeing by incorporating wellness services such as nutrition counseling, massage therapy, and mental health support. This shift acknowledges that overall health extends beyond physical fitness and includes mental and emotional aspects.

Emphasis on Community and Social Connection: Today's fitness gyms prioritize community and social connection. Group fitness classes, team workouts, and fitness challenges foster a sense of belonging and mutual support. This community-focused approach recognizes the motivational power of shared goals and experiences, making the fitness journey more enjoyable and sustainable.

Integration of Digital Platforms: The digital age has brought about a new era in fitness with the integration of online platforms. Virtual workouts, fitness apps, and live streamed classes have become integral parts of the fitness landscape. This allows individuals to access training programs and connects with fitness communities globally, offering flexibility in how and where they pursue their fitness goals.

In conclusion, the evolution of fitness gyms is a dynamic narrative reflecting the changing needs and aspirations of individuals seeking to lead healthier lives. From ancient gymnasiums to high-tech, community-oriented fitness centers, the journey highlights the enduring human pursuit of physical wellbeing and the recognition that fitness is a multifaceted endeavor encompassing mind, body, and community. As we continue into the future, the evolution of fitness gyms is likely to persist, adapting to emerging technologies and evolving societal attitudes towards health and wellness.

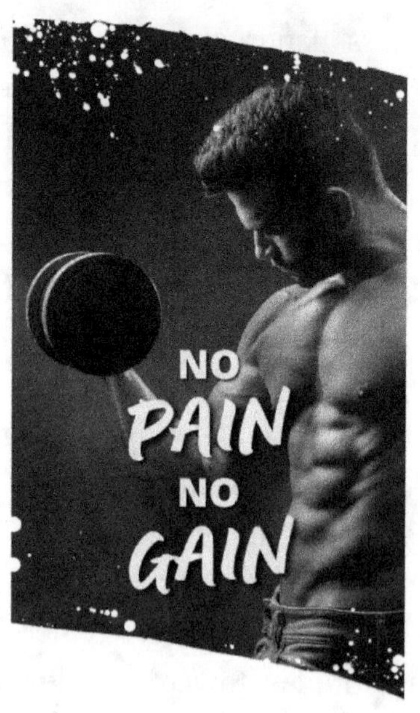

Setting Your Fitness Goals

Setting fitness goals is a crucial step in embarking on a journey toward a healthier and more active lifestyle. Defining personal fitness objectives provides a roadmap for individuals, guiding them through tailored workouts and lifestyle changes. In this exploration of "Defining Personal Fitness Objectives," we delve into the significance of goal setting, the various types of fitness goals, and strategies for creating realistic and sustainable objectives.

Defining Personal Fitness Objectives

The Significance of Goal Setting: Setting clear and specific fitness goals is like plotting coordinates on a map; it gives direction and purpose to your fitness journey. Whether you are a seasoned athlete or a beginner taking the first steps towards a healthier lifestyle, establishing objectives provides a framework for progress and a tangible measure of success.

Understanding Different Types of Fitness Goals: Fitness goals can be broadly categorized into various types, each addressing specific aspects of wellbeing. These categories may include:

Cardiovascular endurance focuses on improving the efficiency of the heart and lungs, often measured by the ability to sustain aerobic activities over an extended period of time.

Strength and Muscle Building: targets enhancing muscle mass, strength, and overall body composition through resistance training exercises. Flexibility and mobility aim to improve the range of motion in joints and enhance overall flexibility, often achieved through stretching and mobility exercises.
Weight management involves goals related to losing, gaining, or maintaining weight, addressing aspects of nutrition, exercise, and lifestyle.
Sport-specific goals: tailored objectives for individuals training for a specific sport or athletic event, focusing on skills, conditioning, and performance improvement.

Goal-setting Techniques: SMART stands for specified, measurable, attainable, relevant, and time-bound. These requirements are often used to create effective fitness goals. With a clear roadmap for monitoring progress, this strategy guarantees that objectives are well-defined and achievable. To illustrate:

Particular: "Lose 10 pounds in three months" is a more targeted aim than the more general "lose weight" one.
Measurable: Quantify your goals to track progress. For instance, "run a 5k in under 30 minutes" is more measurable than simply aiming to "run faster."

Achievable: Set goals that are challenging but attainable based on your current fitness level and circumstances.

Relevant: Ensure your goals align with your overall wellbeing and lifestyle. A relevant goal could be "improve core strength for better posture" if you spend long hours at a desk.

Time-limited.: Decide on a deadline for accomplishing your objectives. This increases urgency and keeps one from putting thing off.

Long-term vs. short-term goals:
Balancing long-term aspirations with short-term milestones is key to sustaining motivation and tracking progress effectively. Long-term goals provide a sense of purpose, while short-term goals offer tangible checkpoints along the way. For example:

Long-term Goal: "Achieve and maintain a healthy weight."

Short-Term Goal: "Lose 2 pounds in the next two weeks by following a balanced diet and exercising three times a week."

Customizing Goals to Individual Needs:
Fitness goals should be personalized, taking into account individual preferences, constraints, and health considerations. What works for one person may not be suitable for another. Tailoring goals to individual needs ensures they are realistic and aligned with lifestyle choices.

Incorporating Variety into Fitness Goals:
Variety is not only the spice of life but also a key ingredient in sustaining interest and motivation in fitness. Incorporating a mix of goals—perhaps focusing on cardiovascular health one month, strength training the next, and flexibility the following—prevents monotony and promotes overall fitness.

Periodic Review and Adjustment:
As your fitness journey progresses, it's essential to periodically review and, if necessary, adjust your goals. Circumstances, priorities, and fitness levels may change, and flexibility in goal setting allows for adaptation without losing sight of the overarching objectives.

Tracking Progress and Celebrating Achievements:
Regularly monitoring progress is a motivating factor in adhering to fitness goals. Tracking can be done through workout logs, fitness apps, or periodic assessments. Celebrating achievements, whether big or small, reinforces positive behavior and keeps the momentum going.

Accountability and Support:
Sharing your fitness goals with a friend, family member, or fitness buddy provides a sense of accountability. Having a support system

encourages adherence to goals, and the shared experience can make the journey more enjoyable.

In conclusion, defining personal fitness objectives is a dynamic and individualized process that goes beyond the surface-level desire for physical change. It involves introspection, a realistic assessment of one's current state of health, and the formulation of goals that align with overall wellbeing. By embracing the SMART criteria, balancing short- and long-term aspirations, and customizing goals to individual needs, individuals can embark on a fitness journey that is not only effective but also sustainable. The evolution of these goals over time, coupled with periodic adjustments, ensures that the fitness journey remains dynamic, engaging, and in tune with the changing needs of the individual. Ultimately, the process of defining and pursuing fitness objectives becomes a transformative and empowering experience, shaping a healthier and more fulfilling lifestyle.

Tailoring workouts for specific goals is the cornerstone of effective and purposeful exercise. Whether aiming for weight loss, muscle gain, improved cardiovascular health, or sport-specific performance, a customized workout plan ensures that each session contributes directly to the desired outcome. In this exploration of "Tailoring Workouts for Specific Goals," we delve into the key principles and strategies to design effective and goal-oriented exercise routines.

Tailoring Workouts for Specific Goals

Identifying Specific Objectives: The first step in tailoring workouts is identifying and understanding the specific fitness goals. This could be anything from shedding excess weight and building muscle to improving endurance or enhancing athletic performance. Each goal requires a distinct approach, emphasizing different aspects of fitness.

Cardiovascular Endurance: For those seeking to improve cardiovascular health and endurance, workouts should prioritize activities that elevate the heart rate over an extended period of time. This could include running, cycling, swimming, or engaging in high-intensity interval training (HIIT). Structuring workouts with intervals of intensity and recovery contributes to cardiovascular adaptations, enhancing overall endurance.

Strength and muscle building: Individuals focused on building strength and muscle mass benefit from resistance training. Tailoring workouts for this goal involves incorporating compound exercises such as squats, dead lifts, and bench presses. Strategic manipulation of sets, reps, and resistance levels is crucial to stimulating muscle growth while allowing for sufficient recovery.

Flexibility and Mobility: Tailoring workouts for improved flexibility and mobility involves integrating stretching and mobility exercises. Incorporating activities like yoga or Pilates enhances range of motion and flexibility. Dynamic stretching before workouts and static stretching in cool-down sessions contribute to improved joint health and overall flexibility.

Weight Management: Those aiming for weight management should combine cardiovascular exercise with strength training. Cardio activities burn calories, while resistance training builds muscle, contributing to an increased metabolic rate. A well-rounded approach also includes a focus on nutrition to create a caloric deficit, aiding in weight loss.

Sport Specific Training: Athletes pursuing sport-specific goals require targeted training that mimics the demands of their chosen sport. This may involve drills, agility exercises, and skill-specific training sessions. Understanding the biomechanics and energy systems relevant to the sport is crucial to tailoring workouts effectively.

Customizing Intensity and Volume: The intensity and volume of workouts play a pivotal role in achieving specific goals. Tailoring these aspects involves manipulating variables like load, repetitions, and rest intervals. Higher intensity and lower repetitions with heavier weights are typical for strength building, while moderate intensity and higher repetitions suit endurance goals.

Periodization: Incorporating per iodization into workout plans is a strategic approach to preventing plateaus and promoting long-term progress. Periodization involves dividing the training into distinct phases, each with a specific focus. For example, a strength-building phase may be followed by a hypertrophy phase, creating a structured progression towards the overall goal.

Consistency and Progress Tracking: Consistency is paramount to achieving any fitness goal. Regularly tracking progress helps adjust workout plans as needed. This could involve recording weights lifted, tracking running times, or monitoring body measurements. Adjustments are made based on the feedback provided by the body's response to the training stimulus.

Balancing cardio and strength training: Many fitness goals benefit from a balanced approach that combines cardiovascular exercise and strength training. This balance ensures a holistic improvement in overall fitness. For instance, someone aiming for weight loss can benefit from burning calories through cardio while simultaneously building lean muscle mass to boost metabolism.

Rest and Recovery: Tailoring workouts also involves considering adequate rest and recovery. Overtraining can hinder progress and increase the risk of injury. Incorporating rest days, proper sleep, and active recovery techniques supports the body's adaptation to the training stimulus.

In conclusion, tailoring workouts for specific goals is a dynamic and personalized process that requires a deep understanding of individual objectives, fitness levels, and preferences. It involves a strategic combination of various exercise modalities, intensity adjustments, and a keen awareness of progress and adaptation. The effectiveness of a tailored workout plan lies not only in its alignment with specific goals but also in its ability to evolve over time. As individuals progress on their fitness journey, ongoing adjustments to the workout routine ensure continued engagement, motivation, and, ultimately, the realization of their desired fitness outcomes.

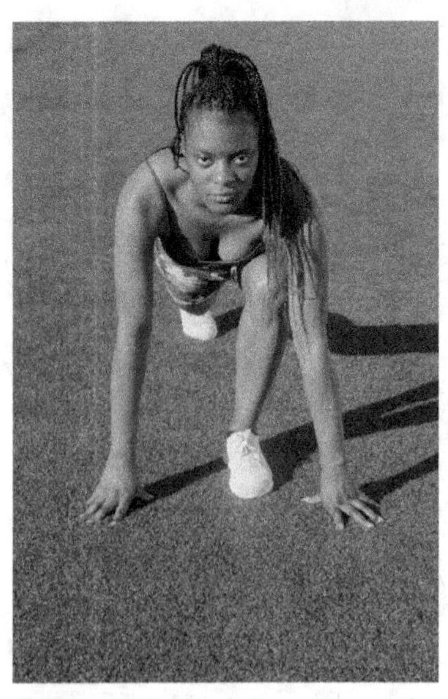

Nutrition for Optimal Performance

Achieving optimal performance, whether in sports, fitness endeavors, or daily life, is closely intertwined with nutrition. The body's ability to function at its best relies heavily on the intake of essential macronutrients—carbohydrates, proteins, and fats. Balancing these macronutrients in your diet is a fundamental aspect of fueling the body for peak performance.

Knowing the Macronutrients:

Carbs: The body uses carbohydrates as its main energy source. They are converted into glucose, which powers a number of biological processes as well as physical endeavors. Complex carbs found in whole grains, fruits, vegetables, and legumes are crucial for optimum performance. They promote endurance throughout longer activities by releasing energy gradually.

The upkeep of bodily tissues and the development and repair of muscles depend heavily on proteins. Athletes and individuals engaged in regular physical activity require an adequate protein intake to support these processes. Sources of lean proteins include poultry, fish, tofu, legumes, and dairy products. The timing of protein intake, especially post exercise, plays a role in optimizing recovery and muscle synthesis.

 Fats: Dietary fats are necessary for the synthesis of hormones and the absorption of fat-soluble vitamins, among other functions of the body. Although fat is often linked to energy storage, it is also an important source of energy for activities that range from mild to moderately intense. A well-balanced diet should include healthy fats such as avocados, nuts, seeds, and olive oil.

The Importance of Balanced Macronutrients:

Energy Balance: Balancing macronutrients ensures that the body receives the right proportion of energy sources. This energy balance is crucial for maintaining weight, whether it's for weight loss, maintenance, or muscle gain. The body's energy needs vary based on factors like age, gender, activity level, and specific performance goals.

Optimal Performance: Athletes, in particular, rely on a balanced intake of macronutrients for optimal performance. Carbohydrates provide quick energy for intense activities, proteins support muscle function and repair, and fats contribute to sustained energy during endurance exercises. Fine-tuning the ratio of these macronutrients can enhance endurance, strength, and overall athletic performance.

Muscle protein synthesis: Protein intake is especially crucial for muscle protein synthesis. Balancing macronutrients ensures that an adequate amount of protein is available to repair and build muscle tissues. This becomes pivotal in scenarios where muscle recovery and growth are integral, such as resistance training or high-intensity workouts.

Satiety and Weight Management: A well-balanced intake of macronutrients contributes to satiety, the feeling of fullness, and satisfaction after eating. This can aid in weight management by preventing overeating and promoting a more mindful approach to food consumption. A diet skewed toward one macronutrient at the expense of others may lead to imbalances and potential health issues.

Blood sugar regulation: Carbohydrates play a significant role in blood sugar regulation. Choosing complex carbohydrates with a lower glycemic index helps maintain steady blood sugar levels, providing a sustained release of energy and preventing energy crashes. This is particularly relevant for activities requiring prolonged endurance.

Strategies for Balancing Macronutrients:

Assessing individual needs: Every individual has unique nutritional requirements based on factors such as age, gender, weight, activity level, and specific fitness goals. Understanding these factors is essential for tailoring macronutrient intake to individual needs.

Meal Timing and Distribution: The distribution of macronutrients throughout the day can impact energy levels and performance. Consuming a balanced meal with a combination of carbohydrates, proteins, and fats before exercise provides fuel, while post-exercise meals support recovery and muscle replenishment. Snacking on nutrient-dense foods between meals can help maintain a steady energy supply.

Carbohydrate Periodization: For athletes engaged in varying intensities of training, carbohydrate periodization involves adjusting carbohydrate intake based on the intensity and duration of workouts. Higher carbohydrate consumption may be beneficial on days with intense training sessions to replenish glycogen stores, while lower intake may be suitable on rest days.

Protein Quality and Quantity: The quality of protein sources and the quantity consumed are both crucial factors. Incorporating a variety of protein-rich foods ensures a spectrum of essential amino acids. Athletes and those engaging in resistance training may benefit from a slightly elevated protein intake to support muscle protein synthesis.

Balancing Fat Intake: Including a variety of healthy fats in the diet is important for overall health. Balancing the intake of omega3 and omega6 fatty acids is beneficial and avoiding excessive consumption of saturated and trans fats supports cardiovascular health. Adjusting fat intake based on energy needs and activity levels is key to maintaining a balanced diet.

Monitoring and Adjusting: Regular monitoring of energy levels, performance, and overall wellbeing can provide valuable feedback on the effectiveness of the macronutrient balance. Adjustments may be necessary based on changes in activity levels, fitness goals, or individual responses to different dietary approaches.

Case Study: Tailoring Macronutrients for Different Goals

Endurance Athlete: Carbohydrates: There is a higher emphasis on complex carbohydrates for sustained energy during long-distance runs or cycling.
Proteins: Adequate protein intake is necessary for muscle repair and recovery.
Fats: Moderate intake for sustained energy; focus on healthy fats.

Strength Trainer:
Carbohydrates: sufficient to fuel workouts, with an emphasis on pre- and post-exercise meals.
Proteins: elevated protein intake to support muscle building and repair.
Fats are adequate for overall health and hormone production.

Weight Loss Seeker: Carbohydrates: Emphasis on complex carbohydrates for sustained energy, but mindful of overall calorie intake.
Proteins are essential for satiety and muscle preservation during weight loss.
Fats: moderate intake, with a focus on healthy fats for satiety.

Conclusion:

Balancing macronutrients in your diet is not a one-size-fits-all approach but rather a personalized journey based on individual needs and goals. Whether striving for optimal athletic performance, weight management, or overall wellbeing, understanding the roles of carbohydrates, proteins, and fats is foundational. The synergy between these macronutrients ensures a holistic approach to nutrition, supporting the body's diverse functions and fueling it for success in various endeavors. Tailoring your macronutrient intake is a dynamic process that requires awareness, flexibility, and a commitment to sustainable, health-promoting dietary practices.

Importance of Hydration in Fitness

Hydration is a cornerstone of overall health, and its significance becomes even more pronounced in the realm of fitness. Whether you're a seasoned athlete, a casual exerciser, or just embarking on a fitness journey, maintaining proper hydration is essential for optimal performance, recovery, and overall wellbeing.

Regulation of Body Temperature: During physical activity, the body temperature rises due to increased metabolic processes. Sweating is the body's natural mechanism to cool down. Proper hydration is crucial for this process, as sweat helps dissipate heat. Insufficient fluid intake can lead to dehydration, impair the body's ability to regulate temperature, and potentially result in heat-related illnesses.

Optimal Physical Performance: Hydration plays a pivotal role in maintaining peak physical performance. Even mild dehydration can lead to a noticeable decline in strength, endurance, and coordination. Athletes and fitness enthusiasts often experience reduced stamina and increased perceived effort when dehydrated. Ensuring adequate fluid intake helps sustain energy levels, allowing for more prolonged and effective workouts.

Electrolyte Balance: Electrolytes, such as sodium, potassium, and magnesium, play a crucial role in nerve function, muscle contractions, and fluid balance within cells. Sweating during exercise results in the loss of electrolytes. Proper hydration with electrolyte fluids, such as sports drinks or coconut water, helps restore and maintain the delicate balance of these essential minerals, preventing issues like muscle cramps and fatigue.

Joint Lubrication and Shock Absorption: Proper hydration is essential for joint health during physical activity. Water serves as a lubricant for joints, facilitating smooth movement and reducing friction. Hydration also contributes to the maintenance of synovial fluid, which cushions joints and aids in shock absorption. Well-lubricated joints are less prone to injuries and perform more efficiently during workouts.

Nutrient Transport and Waste Removal: Water is a fundamental component in the transport of nutrients and the removal of waste products from cells. During exercise, muscles generate metabolic byproducts that need to be efficiently eliminated. Hydration supports the circulatory system in transporting oxygen and nutrients to working muscles while aiding in the removal of waste products like lactic acid. This process is vital for reducing muscle soreness and enhancing recovery.

Cognitive Function and Focus: Dehydration can adversely affect cognitive function and concentration. Even mild dehydration may lead to fatigue, impaired memory, and reduced alertness. In a fitness setting, maintaining mental clarity and focus is crucial for proper form, technique, and overall workout effectiveness. Staying well hydrated ensures that both the body and mind are functioning optimally during exercise.

Preventing Dehydration-Related Complications:

Severe dehydration can lead to serious complications, such as heatstroke, heat exhaustion, or kidney issues. These conditions pose significant health risks and can be especially prevalent during intense or prolonged exercise, particularly in hot and humid conditions. Consistent hydration helps mitigate these risks and contributes to overall safety during physical activity.

Individual hydration needs: Hydration needs are highly individual and depend on various factors, including body weight, climate, exercise intensity, and personal health conditions. Drinking 17–20 ounces of water two hours before doing out, 8 ounces 20–30 minutes beforehand, and 7–10 ounces every 10–20 minutes while working out is advised by the American Council on Exercise. Refueling after exercise is also essential to replace lost fluids.

Signs of dehydration: Recognizing the signs of dehydration is crucial to maintaining optimal fitness. Symptoms include dark yellow urine, thirst, dry mouth, dizziness, fatigue, and reduced urine output. Monitoring these signs during and after exercise helps individuals adjust their hydration practices to meet their specific needs.

Hydration Strategies:

PreHydration: Start your workout or activity well hydrated by consuming fluids throughout the day. This provides a baseline for maintaining proper hydration during exercise.

During Exercise: Regularly sip fluids during exercise, aiming to replace approximately the amount lost through sweat. Water is generally suitable for moderate activities, while longer or more intense workouts may benefit from electrolyte drinks.

Post-Exercise Hydration: Rehydrate after exercise to replace fluid losses. Including a source of electrolytes can be beneficial, especially after prolonged or intense activities.

Monitor Hydration Status: Pay attention to urine color and frequency. Dark yellow urine may indicate dehydration, but light yellow pee usually suggests sufficient hydration.

Adapt to Environmental Conditions: Hydration needs vary based on environmental factors such as temperature and humidity. Adjust your fluid intake accordingly to account for increased sweat rates.

Conclusion:

In the realm of fitness, hydration is not just a matter of quenching thirst; it is a critical component of optimizing performance, supporting recovery, and safeguarding overall health. Whether you're engaged in high-intensity workouts or moderate activities, recognizing the importance of hydration and implementing sound practices ensures that your body functions at its best, helping you achieve your fitness goals safely and effectively.

Effective Cardiovascular Workouts

Cardiovascular exercise is a cornerstone of overall fitness, contributing to heart health, weight management, and endurance. Within the realm of cardiovascular workouts, **the efficacy and efficiency of high-intensity interval training (HIIT) have led to its great popularity.** In this investigation, we examine the fundamentals of HIIT, its advantages, and how to apply this dynamic training strategy to your exercise regimen.

Training with High-Intensity Periods (High-Intensity Interval Training)

The basic idea behind high-intensity interval training (HIIT) is to alternate brief bursts of high-intensity exercise with rest or lower-intensity activities. The idea is to force the body to perform at or near full capacity during the intensive intervals and then take short rest intervals in between. The whole exercise is spent repeating this loop.

Structure of a HIIT Workout: A typical HIIT session involves a warm-up, followed by several rounds of intense intervals and rest or low-intensity recovery periods. The workout concludes with a cool-down. The ratio of work to rest can vary, but a common structure is a 1:1 ratio, such as 30 seconds of intense exercise followed by 30 seconds of rest.

Versatility of Exercises: HIIT is highly versatile and can incorporate a wide range of exercises, including cardiovascular activities like sprinting, cycling, and jumping jacks, as well as strength-training moves like squats, burpees, or pushups. This versatility allows individuals to tailor HIIT workouts based on their fitness level, preferences, and available equipment.

HIIT's advantages

1. One of the main benefits of HIIT is its efficiency in terms of saving time. In comparison to conventional steady-state cardio, the intensity of the exercise enables people to gain significant cardiovascular benefits in a shorter length of time.

2. Caloric Burn and Weight Administration: The vigorous intervals increase metabolism and heart rate, which increases the amount of calories burned both during and

after the exercise. For weight control and fat reduction, this may be helpful.

3. Enhanced Heart Function, Lower Blood Pressure, and Better Cholesterol Profiles: Research has shown that HIIT enhances heart function and improves cardiovascular health. The heart is pushed to its limits during the severe periods, which eventually leads to beneficial changes.

4. Increased Endurance Regular incorporation of HIIT into a fitness routine can contribute to improved endurance. The alternating nature of the workout challenges both aerobic and anaerobic energy systems, enhancing overall stamina.

5. Metabolic Benefits: HIIT has been associated with improved insulin sensitivity and increased fat oxidation. These metabolic benefits are particularly relevant for individuals aiming to manage blood sugar levels and improve overall metabolic health.

7. Adaptability to Various Fitness Levels: HIIT workouts can be modified to accommodate different fitness levels. Beginners may start with shorter, less intense intervals and gradually progress as their fitness improves.

8. PostExercise Oxygen Consumption (EPOC): HIIT induces a phenomenon known as excess post exercise oxygen consumption (EPOC); this means the body continues to burn calories at an elevated rate even after the workout has concluded, contributing to additional energy expenditure.

Safety Considerations: While HIIT offers numerous benefits, it's essential to approach it with caution, especially for individuals with certain health conditions. A proper warm-up is crucial, and beginners may need to start with lower-intensity intervals. Consulting with a healthcare professional or fitness expert before starting a HIIT program is advisable, especially for those with cardiovascular issues or other health concerns.

Sample HIIT Workout: Here's a simple bodyweight HIIT workout that can be done virtually anywhere:

Warm-up (5 minutes): jumping jacks, jogging in place, dynamic stretch.
Intense Interval (30 seconds): Burpees.
Rest or Low-Intensity Interval (30 seconds): march in place or walk.
Intense Interval (30 seconds): High knees.
Rest or Low-Intensity Interval (30 seconds): Side-to-side lunges.
Repeat this cycle for 20–30 minutes.
Cool down (5 minutes): gentle stretches and controlled breathing.

Conclusion:

High-intensity interval training is a powerful addition to any fitness regimen, offering a time-efficient and effective way to improve cardiovascular health, burn calories, and boost overall fitness. The adaptability of HIIT makes it suitable for various fitness levels, and its versatility ensures that workouts remain engaging and challenging. As with any exercise program, safety is paramount, and individuals are encouraged to tailor HIIT to their fitness levels, listen to their bodies, and seek professional guidance when needed. Incorporating HIIT into your routine can unlock a new dimension of cardiovascular fitness, promoting both physical health and exercise enjoyment.

Cardiovascular machines and their benefits

Cardiovascular exercise is a vital component of a well-rounded fitness routine, contributing to heart health, weight management, and overall wellbeing. Cardiovascular machines offer a convenient and controlled environment for individuals to engage in aerobic activities. In this exploration of cardiovascular machines and their benefits, we will delve into the advantages of using machines such as treadmills, elliptical trainers, stationary bikes, and rowing machines.

Treadmills:

Benefits: Versatility: Treadmills allow users to walk, jog, or run at various speeds and inclines. This versatility makes them suitable for individuals at different fitness levels.

Caloric Burn: Running or walking on a treadmill can lead to a significant caloric burn, aiding in weight management and cardiovascular health.

Controlled Environment: Treadmills provide a controlled and cushioned surface, reducing the impact on joints compared to outdoor running.

Programmable Workouts: Many treadmills come with preprogrammed workouts, allowing users to follow specific routines for targeted fitness goals.

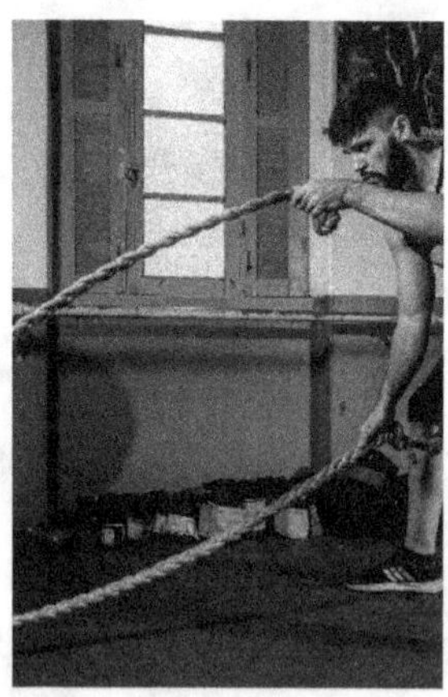

Benefits: minimal impact: The minimal impact of elliptical trainers makes them a good choice for anyone who has joint problems or is looking for a more mild form of training.

Dual Action: As an exercise that works the whole body, the elliptical motion targets different muscle groups and involves the upper and lower body.

Variable Resistance: People may customize the intensity of their exercises using elliptical trainers, as many of them include resistance levels that can be adjusted.

Reverse Motion: Users of some elliptical machines may target various muscle groups and add diversity to their exercises by using the reverse motion option.

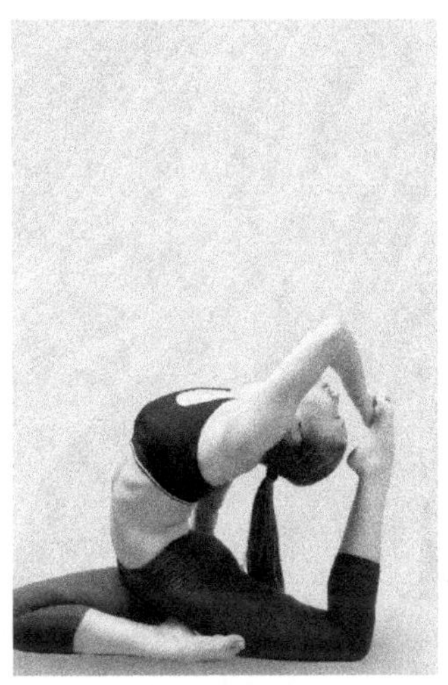

Stationary Bikes:

Benefits: Low Impact: Stationary bikes are gentle on the joints, making them suitable for individuals with arthritis or joint concerns.

Cardiovascular Health: Cycling on a stationary bike is an effective way to improve cardiovascular health, enhance endurance, and boost stamina.

Programmable Resistance: Most stationary bikes allow users to adjust resistance levels, simulating different terrains and intensities.

Comfortable Seating: Many stationary bikes come with adjustable and comfortable seating, promoting longer workout sessions.

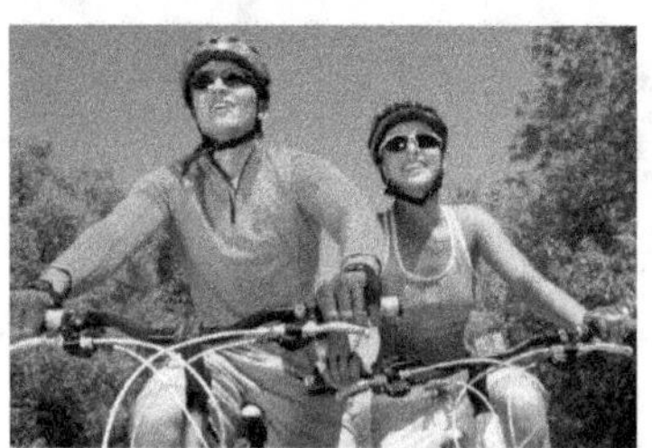

Rowing Machines:

Advantages: Whole-body exercise: By working out various muscle groups, rowing machines provide a thorough full-body exercise that targets the arms, legs, back, and core.

Low Impact: As a low-impact workout, rowing is good for a variety of fitness levels and is easy on the joints.
Cardiovascular Conditioning: Rowing promotes cardiovascular conditioning, improving heart health and lung capacity.

Caloric Burn: Rowing can contribute to effective calorie burning, making it beneficial for weight management.

Stair Climbers:

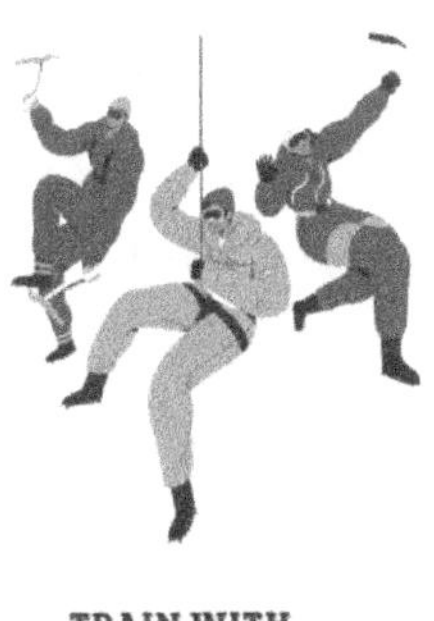

Benefits: Lower Body Engagement: Stair climbers primarily engage the lower body muscles, including the quadriceps, hamstrings, and glutes.

Cardiovascular Intensity: Climbing stairs provides an intense cardiovascular workout, elevating the heart rate and improving cardiovascular fitness.

Caloric Expenditure: Stair climbers can contribute to significant caloric expenditure, aiding in weight loss or maintenance.

Variable Resistance: Many stair climbers allow users to adjust resistance levels, providing options for different fitness levels.

Choosing the Right Cardiovascular Machine:

The selection of a cardiovascular machine depends on individual preferences, fitness goals, and any existing health considerations. Considerations such as impact on joints, full-body engagement, variety of workouts, and programmable features can guide the choice of a suitable machine.

Conclusion:

Cardiovascular machines offer a convenient and controlled means for individuals to engage in aerobic exercises, contributing to improved heart health, weight management, and overall fitness. The variety of machines available allows users to tailor their workouts based on personal preferences and fitness goals. Whether walking on a treadmill, striding on an elliptical, cycling on a stationary bike, rowing, or climbing stairs, these machines provide versatile options for individuals at various fitness levels. Incorporating cardiovascular machine workouts into a well-rounded fitness routine enhances overall physical health and contributes to a sustainable and enjoyable approach to exercise.

Strength Training Essentials: The Basics of Weightlifting

Strength training is a fundamental component of a well-rounded fitness routine, promoting muscle development, increased metabolism, and overall functional fitness. At the core of strength training lies weightlifting, a versatile and effective method for building strength and muscle mass. In this exploration of the basics of weightlifting, we'll delve into the essential principles, techniques, and benefits that form the foundation of this powerful form of exercise.

Weightlifting or resistance Training is the process of challenging and promoting muscular development with the use of external resistance. A variety of equipment, including weight machines, resistance bands, dumbbells, and barbells, as well as body weight exercises, may provide resistance.

Weightlifting Principles: Progressive Overload: The fundamental idea behind weightlifting is progressive overload. To continuously test the muscles, it entails progressively raising the resistance or intensity of the activities. Over time, this process promotes muscular development and adaptation.

Correct Form: Keeping your form correct while lifting weights is essential for efficiency and injury avoidance. By ensuring that the appropriate muscles are used, proper form lowers the possibility of straining joints and supporting systems.

Reps and Sets: Exercises are usually done in sets and repetitions, or reps. A set is a collection of repetitions, and a repetition is one whole exercise action. Individual fitness objectives determine the number of sets and repetitions; for strength and muscular endurance, fewer reps and greater weights are used; for strength, higher reps are used.

Rest and Recovery: Adequate rest between sets and workouts is essential for recovery. Muscles need time to repair and grow stronger. Overtraining without sufficient recovery can lead to fatigue, decreased performance, and an increased risk of injury.

Types of weightlifting exercises:

Compound Exercises: These involve multiple muscle groups and joints working synergistically. Examples include squats, dead lifts, and bench presses. Compound exercises are efficient for targeting multiple muscles in a single movement.

Isolation Exercises: this focus on a specific muscle or muscle group. Examples include bicep curls, tricep extensions, and leg curls. Isolation exercises are useful for targeting and strengthening specific muscles.

Free Weights vs. Machines: Free weights (dumbbells and barbells) provide a greater range of motion and engage stabilizing muscles. Weight machines, on the other hand, offer stability and can be beneficial for beginners or individuals recovering from injuries.

Benefits of weightlifting:

Muscle Development: Weightlifting promotes the development of lean muscle mass, contributing to improved strength, power, and overall muscle tone.

Metabolism Boost: Muscle tissue is metabolically active, meaning it burns more calories at rest than fat tissue. Weightlifting helps increase muscle mass, thereby boosting metabolism and aiding in weight management.

Bone Health: Weightlifting is a weight-bearing activity that stimulates bone density, reducing the risk of osteoporosis and promoting overall bone health.

Functional Fitness: Strength training enhances functional fitness, improving the ability to perform daily activities with ease and reducing the risk of injuries related to muscle imbalances.

Joint Health: Properly executed weightlifting exercises can contribute to joint stability and health. Strengthening the muscles around joints provides support and reduces the risk of injuries.

Mental Health: Regular weightlifting can have positive effects on mental wellbeing. The sense of accomplishment, increased confidence, and release of endorphins contribute to improved mood and reduced stress.

Getting Started with Weightlifting:

Warm-up: Always start with a dynamic warm-up to increase blood flow and prepare muscles for the upcoming workout. Dynamic stretches and light cardio can be effective components of a warm-up.

Start with the basics: Beginners should begin with foundational exercises that target major muscle groups. Squats, lunges, chest presses, and rows are excellent starting points.

Proper Equipment: If using free weights, ensure you have the appropriate equipment, such as a sturdy bench, barbells, and dumbbells. When using weight machines, familiarize yourself with the proper adjustments and settings.

Gradual Progression: Begin with a weight that allows for proper form and execution. As you become comfortable with the exercises, gradually increase the resistance to continue challenging your muscles.

Listen to your body: Pay attention to your body's signals. If you experience pain (not to be confused with the discomfort of a challenging workout), it's essential to address it and, if necessary, seek guidance from a fitness professional or healthcare provider.

Conclusion:

The basics of weightlifting form the cornerstone of a successful strength training program. By understanding and applying the principles of progressive overload, proper form, and varied exercise selection, individuals can embark on a journey of increased strength, muscle development, and overall improved physical wellbeing. Incorporating weightlifting into a well-rounded fitness routine offers numerous benefits, supporting not only physical health but also mental and functional aspects of daily life. As with any exercise program, individuals are encouraged to start gradually, listen to their bodies, and seek guidance from fitness professionals if needed.

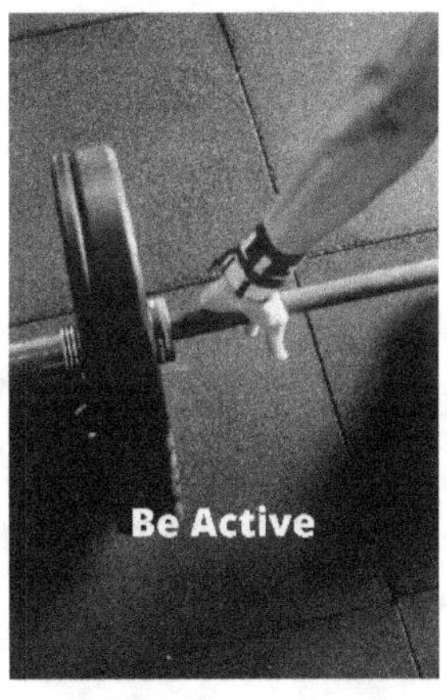

Incorporating Resistance Training: A Path to Strength and Fitness

Resistance training, often synonymous with strength training, is a powerful and versatile exercise modality that involves working against an opposing force to build muscle strength, endurance, and overall fitness. Whether using free weights, resistance bands, or body weight, incorporating resistance training into your fitness routine yields a myriad of benefits. In this exploration of resistance training, we'll delve into the principles, methods, and advantages that make it an indispensable component of a comprehensive exercise program.

Progressive Overload: The fundamental principle of progressive overload applies to resistance training. To stimulate muscle growth and strength gains, it's essential to gradually increase the intensity or resistance over time. This can be achieved by adding weight, adjusting resistance bands, or progressing to more challenging bodyweight exercises.

Specificity: Resistance training should be specific to individual goals. Whether aiming for increased muscle size (hypertrophy), enhanced strength, or muscular endurance, tailoring the resistance training program to align with specific objectives optimizes results.

Variety and Periodization: Incorporating variety into resistance training prevents plateaus and enhances overall fitness. Periodization, the systematic planning of training phases, allows for the manipulation of variables such as intensity, volume, and exercise selection to promote continuous adaptation and progress.

Proper Form: Maintaining proper form during resistance exercises is paramount. It ensures that the targeted muscles are engaged, reducing the risk of injury and maximizing the effectiveness of the workout. If you are unsure about the form, seeking guidance from a fitness professional is advisable.

Methods of resistance training:

Free Weights: Dumbbells, barbells, and kettle bells are classic free-weight options. They engage stabilizing muscles and provide a versatile range of exercises, including squats, dead lifts, and overhead presses.

Resistance Bands: Elastic bands offer variable resistance and are excellent for targeting muscles throughout the entire range of motion. They are portable, suitable for various fitness levels, and can be incorporated into a wide array of exercises.

Bodyweight Exercises: Exercises like pushups, squats, lunges, and planks use the body's own weight as resistance. Bodyweight training enhances functional strength and is accessible for individuals with minimal equipment.

Weight Machines: Weight machines are beneficial for beginners and those targeting specific muscle groups. They provide stability and guide proper movement patterns.

Benefits of Resistance Training:

Muscle Development: Resistance training promotes the growth and development of skeletal muscles, contributing to increased strength and enhanced muscle tone.

Metabolic Boost: Muscle tissue is metabolically active, meaning it burns more calories at rest. Resistance training elevates metabolism, aiding in weight management and fat loss.

Bone Health: Weight bearing exercises, inherent in resistance training, stimulate bone density and contribute to overall bone health, reducing the risk of osteoporosis.

Improved Joint Health: Strengthening muscles around joints enhances joint stability and reduces the risk of injuries or conditions such as arthritis.

Functional Fitness: Resistance training improves overall functional fitness, enhancing the ability to perform daily activities and reducing the risk of muscle imbalances.

Mental Health Benefits: Engaging in regular resistance training has positive effects on mental wellbeing. The sense of accomplishment, improved self-esteem, and release of endorphins contribute to reduced stress and enhanced mood.

Incorporating Resistance Training into Your Routine:

Set clear goals: Define specific and measurable goals for your resistance training program, whether it's building strength, increasing muscle size, or improving muscular endurance.

Start Gradually: If you are new to resistance training, begin with a weight or resistance level that allows for proper form. Focus on mastering fundamental movements before progressing to more complex exercises.

Include Variety: Vary your resistance training routine to prevent monotony and stimulate different muscle groups. This can involve changing exercises, altering intensity, or incorporating different resistance modalities.

Prioritize Recovery: Allow sufficient time for muscles to recover between resistance workouts. This may involve alternating muscle groups on different days or incorporating rest days into your routine.

Seek professional guidance: If uncertain about where to start or how to progress, consider seeking guidance from a certified fitness professional. They can provide personalized advice, ensure proper form, and create a tailored program aligned with your goals.

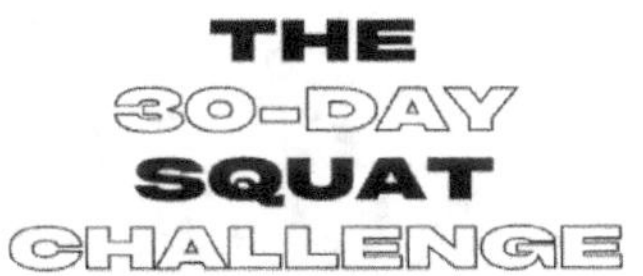

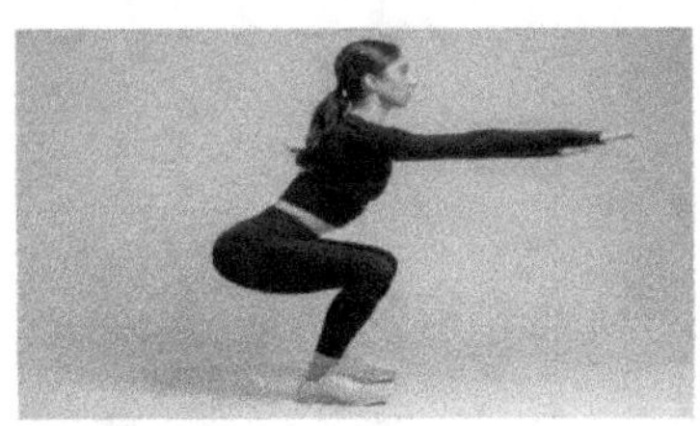

Conclusion:

Incorporating resistance training into your fitness routine is a key pathway to enhanced strength, improved body composition, and overall wellbeing. The principles of progressive overload, specificity, and variety guide effective resistance training programs. Whether using free weights, resistance bands, body weight, or machines, the versatility of resistance training makes it accessible for individuals at various fitness levels. As with any exercise program, it's crucial to start gradually, prioritize proper form, and tailor the routine to align with individual goals. By embracing the power of resistance training, individuals can embark on a transformative journey to greater strength, vitality, and lasting fitness.

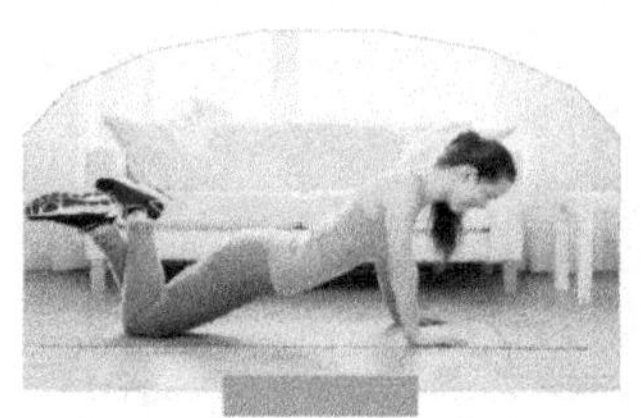

Flexibility and Mobility Exercises: The Foundation of Functional Movement

Flexibility and mobility are integral components of physical fitness, contributing to overall health, injury prevention, and functional movement. Flexibility refers to the range of motion in a joint or group of joints, while mobility encompasses the ability to move a joint through its full range of motion actively. Incorporating flexibility and mobility exercises into your fitness routine fosters joint health, enhances performance, and supports a balanced, functional body. In this exploration, we'll delve into the importance, principles, and examples of flexibility and mobility exercises.

Importance of Flexibility and Mobility:

Injury Prevention: Adequate flexibility and mobility reduce the risk of injuries by allowing joints to move freely through their intended range. Well-maintained joints are less prone to strains, sprains, and other musculoskeletal issues.

Improved Posture: Flexibility and mobility exercises contribute to better posture by promoting optimal alignment of the musculoskeletal system. This, in turn, reduces the risk of discomfort and pain associated with poor posture.

Enhanced Performance: Athletes and fitness enthusiasts benefit from improved performance through an increased range of motion. Whether in sports, weightlifting, or everyday activities, enhanced flexibility and mobility translate to better movement patterns and efficiency.

Functional Movement: Flexibility and mobility exercises support functional movement patterns necessary for daily activities. Tasks like bending, reaching, and twisting become more efficient and less taxing on the body.

Joint Health: Regular flexibility and mobility work helps maintain joint health by preventing stiffness and promoting synovial fluid circulation. This is particularly important for joints that undergo repetitive stress.

Principles of Flexibility and Mobility Exercises:

Dynamic and static stretching: Dynamic stretching involves controlled movements that take joints through their full range of motion. This is ideal for warming up before an activity. Static stretching, where a muscle is lengthened and held for a period of time, is more suitable for cool downs and improving overall flexibility.

Consistency: Flexibility and mobility gains come with consistent practice. Regularly incorporating exercises into your routine ensures that you maintain and gradually improve your range of motion over time.

Balanced Approach: Address all major muscle groups and joints in your flexibility and mobility routine. A balanced approach ensures that no area is neglected, promoting overall functional movement.

Breathing and Relaxation: Incorporate deep breathing and relaxation techniques during flexibility exercises. This helps release tension in muscles and supports a more effective stretch.

Progression: As with other aspects of fitness, progression is key. Gradually increase the intensity and duration of your flexibility and mobility exercises to continue challenging your body and promoting further gains.

Examples of Flexibility and Mobility Exercises:

Dynamic Stretching Routine:

Leg Swings: Forward and sideways leg swings to engage hip flexors and abductors.

Arm Circles: Circulate arms in both directions to warm up shoulder joints.

Torso Twists: Gentle twists to engage the spine and promote flexibility.

Static Stretching Routine: Hamstring Stretch: Seated or standing, reach toward toes to stretch hamstrings.

Hip Flexor Stretch: Kneel in the lunge position to stretch hip flexors.

Chest Opener: Clasp hands behind the back and open the chest for shoulder flexibility.

Mobility Exercises:
Shoulder Circles: Move shoulders in circular motions to enhance shoulder mobility.
Bodyweight Squats: Deep squats promote hip and ankle mobility.
Cat Cow Stretch: a yoga-inspired movement to improve spinal mobility.

Foam Rolling: Foam rolling the calves, quadriceps, and back helps release tension and improve flexibility by targeting the fascia surrounding muscles.

Yoga and Pilates: Yoga: Incorporating yoga into your routine provides a holistic approach to flexibility, mobility, and overall wellbeing. Yoga poses focus on flexibility, balance, and strength, promoting a mind-body connection.

Pilates: Pilate's exercises emphasize core strength, stability, and flexibility. The controlled movements in Pilates enhance overall mobility while targeting specific muscle groups.

Tips for effective flexibility and mobility training:

Warm-up: Always begin flexibility and mobility sessions with a proper warm-up to increase blood flow to the muscles and prepare them for stretching.

Listen to Your Body: Stretch to the point of tension, not pain. Listen to your body's signals and avoid pushing into discomfort.

Include Variety: Rotate through different flexibility and mobility exercises to ensure a comprehensive approach. Variety helps address multiple planes of movement.

Incorporate proprioceptive exercises. Proprioception involves awareness of one's body in space. Exercises like balance work and stability training enhance proprioception, supporting overall movement quality.

Conclusion:

Flexibility and mobility exercises are the foundation of a well-rounded fitness routine, promoting joint health, injury prevention, and functional movement. Whether you're an athlete looking to enhance performance or someone aiming for overall wellbeing, incorporating dynamic and static stretching, mobility exercises, and mind-body practices like yoga can significantly contribute to your fitness journey. The principles of consistency, balance, and progression guide effective flexibility and mobility training, ensuring that you maintain and continually improve your range of motion for a healthier and more functional body.

Dynamic vs. Static Stretching:

Dynamic stretching involves controlled, active movements that take joints and muscles through their full range of motion. Unlike static stretching, where a position is held for an extended period, dynamic stretching is more fluid and incorporates movements that mimic activities you might perform during your workout or daily life. This type of stretching is particularly beneficial as part of a warm-up routine.

Benefits of Dynamic Stretching:

Increased Blood Flow: Dynamic stretching elevates your heart rate and increases blood flow to your muscles, preparing them for more intense activity.

Improved Flexibility: Performing dynamic stretches actively engages your muscles and gradually increases your range of motion over time.

Enhanced Joint Mobility: Dynamic stretching targets multiple joints simultaneously, promoting better joint mobility and overall flexibility.

Neuromuscular Activation: The controlled movements in dynamic stretching stimulate the nervous system, enhancing the connection between your muscles and brain.

Warming up Muscles: Dynamic stretching warms up your muscles, making them more pliable and ready for the dynamic movements involved in various activities.

Common Dynamic Stretching Exercises:

Leg Swings: Forward and sideways leg swings dynamically engage the hip flexors and abductors.

Arm Circles: Circulating your arms in both directions warms up the shoulder joints and improves flexibility.

Torso Twists: Gentle twists from side to side engage the spine, promoting flexibility and warming up the core.

High Knees: Lifting your knees towards your chest dynamically engages the hip flexors and quadriceps.

Jumping jacks are a full-body movement involving arm and leg coordination, promoting overall flexibility and increasing heart rate.

Static Stretching: The Art of Holding Positions

Static stretching involves lengthening a muscle to the point of mild discomfort and holding the position for an extended period, typically ranging from 15 to 60 seconds. This type of stretching is often performed after a workout or as part of a cool-down routine. The aim is to increase flexibility and promote relaxation in targeted muscle groups.

Benefits of Static Stretching:

Improved Flexibility: Holding a stretch allows the muscle fibers and connective tissue to gradually elongate, contributing to improved flexibility.

Enhanced Range of Motion: Static stretching helps increase the range of motion around specific joints, making movements smoother and more controlled.

Relaxation and Stress Reduction: The prolonged, gentle nature of static stretching promotes relaxation, reduces muscle tension, and contributes to stress reduction.

Muscle Recovery: Performing static stretches after a workout can aid in muscle recovery by reducing muscle soreness and promoting blood flow.

Joint Alignment: Static stretching can help improve joint alignment, particularly when focusing on muscle groups that influence joint stability.

Common static stretching exercises:

Hamstring Stretch: Seated or standing, reaching toward your toes stretches the hamstrings.

Hip Flexor Stretch: Kneeling in lunge position elongates the hip flexors.

Chest Opener: Clasping hands behind the back and opening the chest enhances shoulder flexibility.

Quadriceps Stretch: Standing or lying down, pulling your heel towards your buttocks stretches the quadriceps.

Calf Stretch: Leaning against a wall with one foot forward stretches the calf muscles.

Choosing the Right Mix:

While both dynamic and static stretching offer unique benefits, the choice between them depends on the context of your workout.

Warm-up: Dynamic stretching is ideal for warming up before more intense physical activity. It prepares your body for dynamic movements, increases blood flow, and actively engages your muscles.

Cool Down: Static stretching is well-suited for the cool down phase after a workout. Holding static stretches when your muscles are warm can help improve flexibility, relax tense muscles, and contribute to overall recovery.

Sports Specificity: Consider the demands of your specific activity. If your workout involves explosive or dynamic movements, dynamic stretching may be more appropriate. For activities requiring sustained flexibility, static stretching is valuable.

Guidelines for Safe Stretching:

Warm-up First: Before engaging in any stretching routine, ensure you warm up your body with light aerobic activity to increase blood flow to the muscles.

Avoid Bouncing: Whether dynamic or static, bouncing during stretches can lead to injury. Maintain a controlled, steady movement.

Breathing: Breathe deeply and consistently during stretches to promote relaxation and enhance the stretch.

Individualize Your Routine: Tailor your stretching routine to your specific needs and the requirements of your chosen physical activities.

Listen to your body: Stretch to the point of mild discomfort, not pain. If you feel pain, ease off the stretch.

Conclusion:

Incorporating both dynamic and static stretching into your fitness routine provides a well-rounded approach to flexibility and mobility. Dynamic stretching primes your body for movement and increases your heart rate, while static stretching contributes to improved flexibility, muscle relaxation, and enhanced recovery. By understanding the benefits and incorporating the right type of stretching at the right time, you can optimize your flexibility and mobility for a more effective and safe workout routine.

Yoga and Pilates for Flexibility

Yoga is a centuries-old practice that integrates physical postures, breath control, and meditation. While yoga offers a holistic approach to wellbeing, it is particularly renowned for enhancing flexibility. The combination of asanas (postures) and mindful breathing fosters a deep connection between the body and mind, promoting not only physical flexibility but also mental resilience.

Benefits of Yoga for Flexibility:

1. Increased Range of Motion: Yoga postures are designed to move joints through their full range, gradually improving flexibility over time.

2. Balanced Flexibility: Yoga encourages flexibility in all directions, promoting balanced development throughout the body.

3. Stress Reduction: The meditative aspect of yoga contributes to stress reduction by allowing muscles to relax and facilitating deeper stretches.

4. Improved Posture: Many yoga poses focus on spinal alignment, contributing to better posture and reduced strain on the musculoskeletal system.

5. Enhanced Body Awareness: Yoga encourages awareness of body sensations, fostering a mindful connection that supports safer and more effective stretching.

Common types of yoga for flexibility:

1. Hatha Yoga is a foundational practice that involves holding poses, emphasizing breath control, and promoting overall flexibility.

2. Vinyasa Yoga: Characterized by flowing sequences, vinyasa yoga incorporates movement with breath, promoting flexibility through dynamic transitions.

3. Yin yoga involves passive, long-held poses that target connective tissues, facilitating deep stretching and enhanced flexibility.

4. Restorative Yoga: Centered on relaxation and gentle stretching, restorative yoga encourages flexibility through supported poses and deep breathing.

5. Ashtanga Yoga: A dynamic and physically demanding style, Ashtanga yoga involves a set sequence of postures, promoting strength, flexibility, and endurance.

6. Iyengar Yoga: Emphasizing precise alignment and the use of props, Iyengar yoga allows for gradual progression in flexibility while ensuring proper form.

Pilates: Core-Centric Flexibility and Strength

Pilates is a low-impact exercise method that focuses on building core strength, stability, and flexibility. Developed by Joseph Pilates, this practice involves controlled movements that emphasize the mind-body connection. Pilates is particularly effective for developing a strong and flexible core, which is essential for overall stability and movement control.

Benefits of Pilates for Flexibility:

1. Core Flexibility: Pilates targets the deep muscles of the core, promoting flexibility and strength in the abdominal, pelvic, and lower back regions.

2. Increased Joint Range: Pilates exercises are designed to work joints through their full range of motion, contributing to overall flexibility.

3. Muscle Lengthening: Many Pilates movements involve controlled muscle lengthening, helping to improve flexibility in various muscle groups.

4. Improved Posture: Pilates emphasizes proper alignment, leading to improved posture and reduced strain on the spine and supporting structures.

5. Enhanced Mind-Body Awareness: Similar to yoga, Pilates encourages a heightened awareness of body movement and breath, fostering a mindful approach to flexibility training.

Common Elements of Pilates for Flexibility:

- Mat Exercises: These involve a series of controlled movements on a mat, targeting core strength and flexibility.

- Reformer Workouts: Pilates reformer machines incorporate resistance through springs, allowing for a wide range of exercises that enhance flexibility and strength.

- Flexibility Specific Movements: Pilates includes specific exercises aimed at increasing flexibility, such as leg circles, spinal twists, and stretches.

- Breath Control: Pilates places emphasis on breath control during exercises, promoting relaxation, and supporting effective stretching.

Choosing Between Yoga and Pilates:

Yoga is ideal for those seeking a holistic practice that encompasses flexibility, mindfulness, and spiritual elements. Yoga offers a diverse range of styles, allowing individuals to find a practice that aligns with their goals and preferences.

Pilates is suitable for individuals focusing on core strength, stability, and overall body conditioning. Pilates is particularly effective for those looking to improve flexibility while emphasizing controlled and precise movements.

Integrating Yoga and Pilates:

1. Combined Benefits: Many individuals find that incorporating elements of both yoga and Pilates into their routine provides a comprehensive approach to flexibility, strength, and overall wellbeing.

2. Balance of Strength and Flexibility: While yoga may emphasize flexibility and mindfulness, Pilates contributes to core strength and stability. Together, they create a

balanced routine that addresses various aspects of physical fitness.

3. Variety in Routine: Combining yoga and Pilates sessions adds variety to your routine, reducing the risk of boredom and engaging different muscle groups through diverse movements.

Guidelines for Practicing Yoga and Pilates:

1. Mindful Practice: Both yoga and Pilates benefit from a mindful approach. Pay attention to your breath, body sensations, and movement patterns.

2. Consistency: Regular practice is key to experiencing the full benefits of yoga and Pilates. Aim for a balanced routine that includes flexibility, strength, and relaxation.

3. Progress Gradually: Flexibility gains take time. Gradually progress in the intensity and duration of poses or exercises, allowing your body to adapt.

4. Listen to your body: Respect your body's limitations and avoid pushing yourself into pain. Discomfort during stretching is normal, but sharp pain should be avoided.

5. Seek professional guidance. If you're new to yoga or Pilates, consider taking classes with certified instructors. They can provide guidance on proper form and ensure that you're practicing safely.

Conclusion:

Yoga and Pilates offer unique paths to flexibility, strength, and overall wellbeing. Whether you choose the holistic and mindful approach of yoga or the core centric strength of Pilates, both practices contribute to increased flexibility through controlled movements and a focus on mind-body connection. The key is to align your choice with your fitness goals, preferences, and the overall balance you seek in your exercise routine. Integrating elements of both yoga and Pilates can provide a well-rounded approach to flexibility training, enhancing not only physical flexibility but also mental and emotional resilience.

Mind-Body Connection in Fitness

Understanding and harnessing the mind-body connection is crucial for achieving optimal fitness and overall wellbeing. The interplay between mental and physical aspects significantly influences performance, recovery, and the overall fitness journey. In this exploration, we'll delve into the significance of the mind-body connection, meditation techniques tailored for athletes, and the role of mental resilience in physical training.

Meditation Techniques for Athletes

Meditation, often associated with calm and introspective practices, has increasingly found its way into the training routines of athletes seeking a competitive edge. Beyond physical prowess, mental fortitude and focus are essential elements for success in any sport. Here, we'll delve into meditation techniques designed specifically for athletes, exploring how these practices enhance concentration, reduce stress, and contribute to overall wellbeing.

Benefits of Meditation for Athletes:

1. improved Concentration: Meditation cultivates the ability to focus the mind, a critical aspect for athletes who need to maintain concentration during training and competitions.

2. Stress Reduction: The demands of athletic training and competition can induce stress. Meditation techniques, particularly mindfulness meditation, have been shown to reduce stress and promote a sense of calm.

3. Enhanced Recovery: Adequate rest and recovery are integral to athletic performance. Meditation, especially practices that encourage relaxation, aids in the recovery process by promoting restful sleep and reducing muscle tension.

4. Emotional Regulation: Athletes often face intense emotions, from pre-competition anxiety to the highs and lows of victory and defeat. Meditation helps in developing emotional resilience and regulation, allowing athletes to navigate the emotional aspects of their journey more effectively.

5. Increased Body Awareness: Meditation encourages a heightened awareness of bodily sensations. This enhanced body awareness can be particularly beneficial for athletes,

helping them tune into their bodies' signals and respond appropriately to prevent injuries.

Meditation Techniques for Athletes:

1. Mindfulness Meditation: Focus on Breath: Athletes can practice mindfulness by focusing on their breath. This involves paying attention to the inhalation and exhalation, bringing the mind back to the breath when distractions arise.

2. Body Scan: Athletes can engage in a body scan, systematically directing attention to different parts of the body, noting sensations, and promoting relaxation.

3. Guided Visualization: Positive Outcome Visualization: Athletes visualize successful outcomes, imagining themselves executing movements flawlessly and achieving their goals. This technique enhances self-confidence and mental preparedness.

4. Performance Enhancement Visualization: Athletes visualize specific aspects of their performance, such as perfect form, speed, or accuracy. This mental rehearsal can positively impact actual physical execution.

5. Transcendental Meditation (TM): In TM, athletes repeat a specific mantra silently. This technique aims to transcend ordinary thought processes, promoting a state of deep rest and relaxation. TM has been associated with reduced stress and improved cognitive function.

6. Movement Based Meditation: Yoga: Integrating yoga postures and breath work into a meditation practice can enhance flexibility, balance, and mindfulness. Yoga provides a holistic approach to both physical and mental well-being.

7. Tai Chi: This martial art involves slow, flowing movements combined with deep breathing. Tai Chi not only enhances physical coordination but also cultivates a meditative state.

8. Focused Attention Meditation: Single-Point Focus: Athletes can choose a specific point of focus, such as a sound, object, or mantra. Concentrating on this focal point helps quiet the mind and build concentration.

9. Breath Counting: Athletes count their breaths, focusing on each inhalation and exhalation. This simple yet effective technique enhances mindfulness and concentration.

Incorporating Meditation into Athletic Training:

- PreCompetition Rituals: Athletes can establish precompetition rituals that include a brief meditation session. This can help calm nerves, enhance focus, and set a positive tone for the upcoming challenge.

- Recovery Sessions: Including meditation in posttraining or postcompetition recovery routines can aid relaxation, reduce muscle tension, and contribute to overall recovery.

- Consistent Practice: Like any skill, the benefits of meditation compound with consistent practice. Athletes are encouraged to integrate meditation into their daily routines to experience its long-term advantages.

- Adapting to Individual Preferences: Meditation is a versatile practice, and athletes may explore various techniques to find what resonates with them. Whether it's guided visualization, mindfulness, or movement-based meditation, adapting to individual preferences enhances engagement.

- Mindful Movement: Combining meditation with movement, such as walking or jogging mindfully, provides athletes with an opportunity to integrate mental focus with physical activity.

The Power of a Resilient Mind in Fitness

Mental resilience, the ability to adapt and bounce back from challenges, is a cornerstone of successful physical training. Beyond physical strength and endurance, cultivating mental toughness is vital for navigating setbacks, pushing through plateaus, and sustaining long-term fitness goals. In this exploration, we'll delve into the significance of mental resilience in physical training, strategies for building mental toughness, and the holistic impact on overall wellbeing.

Importance of Mental Resilience in Fitness:

Navigate Setbacks: Fitness journeys are rarely linear. Individuals encounter plateaus, injuries, or periods of low motivation. Mental resilience equips individuals to navigate setbacks, learn from challenges, and stay committed to their goals.

Overcome Plateaus: Plateaus, where progress seems to stall, are a common aspect of fitness. Mental resilience encourages individuals to reassess their approach, make necessary adjustments, and persist through plateaus.

Manage Stress: Physical training can be demanding, leading to stress on both the body and mind. Mental resilience assists individuals in managing stress, preventing burnout, and maintaining a balanced approach to training.

Sustain Motivation: Motivation can fluctuate, especially during extended fitness journeys. Mental resilience provides the fortitude to stay motivated, set new goals, and find intrinsic sources of inspiration.

Embrace Consistency: Long-term fitness success is rooted in consistency. Mental resilience helps individuals establish sustainable habits, navigate disruptions, and prioritize their wellbeing consistently.

Strategies for Building Mental Resilience:

Goal Setting and Reframing: Clear Objectives: Clearly define short-term and long-term fitness goals. This clarity provides a roadmap and a sense of purpose.

Reframing Challenges: View challenges as opportunities for growth rather than insurmountable obstacles. Reframing perspectives fosters a resilient mindset.

Adaptability and Flexibility: Adjusting Expectations: Recognize that flexibility is a strength. Be open to adjusting expectations and adapting goals based on evolving circumstances.

Learn from Setbacks: Instead of viewing setbacks as failures, approach them as opportunities to learn and refine your approach. Each challenge is a chance for growth.

Mindfulness Practices: Present Moment Awareness: Mindfulness practices, such as meditation and mindful breathing, cultivate present-moment awareness. This helps individuals focus on the task at hand rather than being overwhelmed by future concerns or past challenges, fostering mental resilience.

Stress Reduction Techniques: Incorporate stress reduction techniques like deep breathing, progressive muscle relaxation, or visualization to manage stressors effectively.

Positive Self Talk: Constructive Language: Replace negative self-talk with positive, constructive language. Encourage yourself, acknowledge progress, and affirm your capabilities.

Affirmations: Develop affirmations that align with your fitness goals. Repeat these positive statements regularly to reinforce a resilient mindset.

Focus on the process. Process-Oriented Goals: Shift the focus from solely outcome-based goals to process-oriented goals. Emphasize the daily habits and behaviors that contribute to long-term success.

Celebrate Small Wins: Acknowledge and celebrate small victories along the way. Recognizing progress, no matter how incremental, sustains motivation.

Cultivate a Growth Mindset: Embrace Challenges: Adopt a growth mindset by viewing challenges as opportunities to develop skills and resilience. Embracing challenges as part of the growth process facilitates a positive perspective.

Learn from Feedback: See feedback, whether from trainers, peers, or personal experiences, as valuable information for improvement. A growth mindset thrives on continuous learning.

Build a supportive network: Community Engagement: Surround yourself with a supportive fitness community. Sharing experiences, successes, and challenges fosters a sense of belonging and resilience.

Professional Guidance: Seek guidance from fitness professionals or coaches who can provide expertise, encouragement, and tailored advice for your fitness journey.

Periodization and Recovery: Strategic Planning: Incorporate periodization into your training plan, allowing for planned variations in intensity and recovery. This strategic approach prevents burnout and supports long-term resilience.

Prioritize Recovery: Recognize the importance of rest and recovery in building mental resilience. Quality sleep, proper nutrition, and active recovery contribute to overall wellbeing.

Visualizations and Mental Rehearsal: Positive Imagery: Engage in positive visualizations where you imagine achieving your fitness goals. This mental rehearsal contributes to confidence and mental resilience.

Mental Rehearsal: Visualize overcoming challenges and executing exercises with precision. This mental rehearsal primes the mind for success during actual physical training.

Holistic Impact on Well-Being:

The cultivation of mental resilience in fitness extends beyond the gym or training space, positively influencing various aspects of overall wellbeing.

- Stress reduction and emotional wellbeing: Mental resilience techniques, such as mindfulness and positive self-talk, contribute to stress reduction and emotional wellbeing. Managing stressors effectively enhances emotional health.

- Improved Decision-making: A resilient mindset supports improved decision-making, both in fitness-related choices and broader life decisions. Clarity of thought and adaptability contribute to sound decision-making.

- Enhanced Coping Skills: Individuals with strong mental resilience develop enhanced coping skills. They can navigate challenges, setbacks, and unexpected events with composure and effectiveness.

- Quality of relationships: The positive mindset cultivated through mental resilience practices extends to relationships. Effective communication, empathy, and adaptability contribute to healthier connections with others.

- Sense of Purpose: The pursuit of fitness goals, coupled with a resilient mindset, provides individuals with a sense of purpose. Having clear objectives and overcoming challenges fosters a meaningful and purpose-driven approach to life.

- A Balanced Approach to Fitness: Mental resilience promotes a balanced approach to fitness. Individuals are more likely to listen to their bodies, avoid extremes, and prioritize overall wellbeing rather than fixating solely on physical outcomes.

- Life Satisfaction: The satisfaction derived from overcoming challenges, achieving fitness milestones, and maintaining a resilient mindset contributes to overall life satisfaction.

Incorporating Mental Resilience into Fitness Routines:

Reflect and set intentions: Regularly reflect on your fitness journey. Acknowledge challenges, celebrate achievements, and set intentions for continued growth.

Daily Mindfulness Practices: Incorporate brief mindfulness practices into your daily routine. This can be as simple as a few minutes of deep breathing or mindful stretching.

Regular Goal Evaluation: Periodically, reassess your fitness goals. Ensure they align with your current aspirations and circumstances. Adjust goals as needed to maintain motivation.

Diversify Training Modalities: Integrate diverse training modalities to keep your routine engaging. Exploring new activities challenges both the body and mind, fostering mental resilience.

Seek professional support. Consider consulting with fitness professionals or mental health practitioners who specialize in sports psychology. Their guidance can provide valuable insights and strategies for building mental resilience.

Connect with a Community: Engage with a fitness community, whether in person or online. Sharing experiences, challenges, and triumphs creates a supportive network that enhances mental resilience.

Celebrate Progress: Regularly celebrate your progress, regardless of scale. Acknowledging the journey and appreciating your efforts contributes to a positive and resilient mindset.

Conclusion:

The mind-body connection in fitness is a dynamic and intricate interplay that goes beyond physical strength and endurance. Meditation techniques tailored for athletes and the cultivation of mental resilience are integral components of a holistic approach to wellbeing. By incorporating mindfulness practices, setting intentions, and developing mental toughness, individuals can enhance their fitness journey, navigate challenges effectively, and sustain long-term wellbeing. The impact of a resilient mindset extends far beyond the gym, positively influencing various aspects of life and contributing to a fulfilling and purpose-driven existence.

Recovery Strategies

Recovery is an often underestimated but fundamental aspect of any fitness journey. The body undergoes stress during workouts, and adaptation and growth occur during periods of rest. In this exploration, we'll emphasize the importance of rest days and delve into the significance of postworkout nutrition for effective recovery.

Importance of Rest Days

In the pursuit of fitness goals, the impulse to push harder and train more frequently can be strong. However, rest days are not a sign of weakness; they are a strategic component of any well-rounded fitness plan. Understanding the importance of rest days involves recognizing the physiological and psychological benefits they offer.

Physiological Benefits of Rest Days:

1. Muscle Repair and Growth: During intense workouts, microscopic damage occurs in muscle fibers. Rest days allow the body to repair and rebuild these fibers, contributing to muscle growth and increased strength.

2. Prevention of overtraining: Overtraining can lead to fatigue, decreased performance, and increased susceptibility to injuries. Adequate rest prevents the negative effects of overtraining, ensuring long-term sustainability in fitness pursuits.

3. Hormonal Balance: Hormones play a crucial role in muscle repair and overall wellbeing. Rest days help maintain a balanced hormonal environment, supporting recovery and minimizing the risk of hormonal imbalances associated with chronic training stress.

4. Immune System Support: Intense and prolonged exercise can temporarily suppress the immune system. Rest days provide an opportunity for the immune system to rebound, reducing the likelihood of illness or infection.

5. Energy Restoration: Physical activity depletes energy stores. Rest days allow for the replenishment of glycogen stores and the restoration of energy levels, ensuring optimal performance during subsequent workouts.

Psychological Benefits of Rest Days:

1. Mental Refreshment: Continuous training can lead to mental fatigue and burnout. Rest days provide an essential mental break, allowing individuals to recharge, regain focus, and approach subsequent workouts with renewed enthusiasm.

2. Reduced stress and anxiety: Exercise is a stressor on the body, and constant exertion without adequate rest can lead to elevated stress levels. Rest days contribute to stress reduction, promoting overall mental wellbeing.

3. Prevention of Exercise Addiction: While exercise is beneficial, excessive training can lead to exercise addiction, which is characterized by an unhealthy obsession with physical activity. Rest days are crucial for preventing the development of this detrimental mindset.

4. Balanced Lifestyle: Incorporating rest days foster a balanced lifestyle. Fitness is just one aspect of wellbeing,

and rest days provide an opportunity to engage in other activities, cultivate hobbies, and spend time with loved ones.

5. Injury Prevention: Continuous strain on muscles and joints without adequate rest increases the risk of injuries. Rest days allow for the recovery of connective tissues and joints, reducing the likelihood of overuse injuries.

Strategies for effective rest days:

- Active Recovery: Engage in low-intensity activities on rest days, such as walking, cycling, or yoga. Active recovery promotes blood flow, aids in muscle recovery, and contributes to overall flexibility.

- Quality Sleep: Sleep is a crucial component of recovery. Aim for 79 hours of quality sleep each night, especially on rest days, to support the body's repair processes.

- Hydration: Proper hydration is essential for recovery. Ensure adequate water intake on rest days to support metabolic processes, joint health, and overall wellbeing.

- Nutrient Rich Diet: Maintain a balanced and nutrient-dense diet on rest days. Adequate protein, carbohydrates, and healthy fats support recovery processes and energy replenishment.

- Self-care Practices: Incorporate self-care practices such as massage, foam rolling, or stretching on rest days. These activities can alleviate muscle tension and enhance overall wellbeing.

- Mindfulness and Relaxation: Engage in mindfulness practices or relaxation techniques on rest days. This can include meditation, deep breathing exercises, or simply taking time to unwind and distress.

The Balance between Consistency and Rest:

While the commitment to consistency is commendable in any fitness journey, it's essential to recognize that progress occurs not only during active training but also during periods of rest. The delicate balance between consistent training and adequate recovery is where sustainable fitness gains are achieved.

1. Individual Variability: The ideal frequency and structure of rest days can vary among individuals. Factors such as age, fitness level, training intensity, and overall health influence the appropriate balance between training and rest.

2. Listening to Your Body: Pay attention to how your body responds to training. Signs of fatigue, persistent soreness, or changes in performance may indicate the need for additional rest or a modification in training intensity.

3. Periodization: Implementing periodization in training plans involves strategically incorporating periods of increased

and decreased intensity. This structured approach optimizes performance and allows for planned periods of rest.

4. Active Monitoring: Regularly assess your energy levels, mood, and overall wellbeing. If you consistently feel fatigued or notice a decline in performance, it may be an indication that adjustments to your training or rest routine are needed.

Rest days are not a concession to weakness; they are a strategic investment in the body's ability to recover, adapt, and thrive. Recognizing the physiological and psychological benefits of rest days is integral to achieving sustainable progress in fitness. Incorporating effective rest day strategies, such as active recovery, quality sleep, and self-care practices, enhances overall wellbeing and contributes to a balanced and successful fitness journey.

Fueling the Gains: The Critical Role of Post-Workout Nutrition:

Post workout nutrition plays a pivotal role in the recovery process, influencing muscle repair, glycogen replenishment, and overall recovery. The body undergoes stress during exercise, depleting energy stores and causing micro tears in muscle fibers. Proper post-workout nutrition provides the necessary nutrients to support the body's recovery and enhance the benefits of physical activity.

Key Components of Post-Workout Nutrition:

Protein: Muscle Repair and Growth: Protein is crucial for muscle repair and growth. During exercise, muscle proteins are broken down, and consuming protein post workout provides the essential amino acids needed for their synthesis.

Optimal Timing: Consuming protein within the first hour after exercise, known as the "anabolic window," is often recommended to maximize muscle protein synthesis.

Sources: Include high-quality protein sources such as lean meats, poultry, fish, eggs, dairy, plant-based proteins, or protein supplements.

Carbohydrates: Glycogen Replenishment: Carbohydrates are the body's primary source of energy. Consuming carbohydrates after a workout helps replenish glycogen stores depleted during exercise, supporting energy levels for subsequent sessions.

Quick Absorption: Fast-digesting carbohydrates, such as those found in fruits or easily digestible grains, are beneficial for quickly replenishing glycogen.

Balanced Ratios: The ratio of protein to carbohydrates in a post workout meal or snack can depend on individual goals, but a common recommendation is a 3:1 or 4:1 ratio of carbohydrates to protein.

Hydration: Rehydration: Sweating during exercise leads to fluid loss, and rehydration is crucial for overall recovery. Consuming water or a rehydration beverage helps restore fluid balance.

Electrolytes: In cases of intense or prolonged exercise, replacing electrolytes (sodium, potassium, and magnesium) lost through sweat is important for maintaining proper cellular function.

Antioxidants: Combating Oxidative Stress: Intense exercise can produce oxidative stress, contributing to muscle damage. Antioxidants, found in fruits and vegetables, help combat oxidative stress and support recovery.

Vitamins C and E: These vitamins, in particular, have been studied for their antioxidant properties and potential benefits in reducing exercise-induced muscle damage.

Timing and frequency: Post Workout Window While the concept of an immediate post workout meal has been emphasized, current research suggests that the overall daily nutrient intake is more important than an exact timing window.

Balanced Meals: Ensuring balanced meals throughout the day that include a combination of protein, carbohydrates, healthy fats, and micronutrients supports overall recovery.

Individualized Considerations:

1. Fitness Goals: Muscle Building: Those aiming to build muscle may benefit from a higher protein intake in their post workout nutrition to support muscle protein synthesis.

2. Endurance Training: Endurance athletes may prioritize carbohydrate intake to replenish glycogen stores for sustained energy during prolonged activities.

3. Dietary Preferences: Plant-Based Options: Individuals following a plant-based diet can obtain postworkout nutrition from sources such as tofu, tempeh, legumes, quinoa, and plant-based protein supplements.

4. Whole Foods vs. Supplements: While supplements can be convenient, whole food sources are often preferred for providing a broader spectrum of nutrients.

5. Health Conditions: Metabolic Conditions: Individuals with specific health conditions, such as diabetes, may need to consider their carbohydrate intake and monitor blood sugar levels post-exercise.

6. Food Sensitivities: Those with food sensitivities or allergies should choose postworkout foods that align with their dietary restrictions.

Practical Tips for Effective Post-Workout Nutrition:

1. Prepare Ahead: Meal Planning: Preparing postworkout meals or snacks in advance ensures that you have a

convenient and nutritionally balanced option readily available.

2. Portable Options: For those with time constraints, portable and easily transportable snacks, such as protein bars or shakes, can be convenient choices.

3. Whole Foods Emphasis: Nutrient-Dense Choices: Prioritize whole, nutrient-dense foods to obtain a wide range of vitamins, minerals, and phytonutrients.

4. Lean Protein Sources: Opt for lean protein sources to minimize unnecessary saturated fats and support muscle repair.

5. Hydration Awareness: Consistent Hydration: Maintaining hydration throughout the day is essential for overall health and aids in the recovery process.

6. Electrolyte Balance: If engaging in intense or prolonged exercise, consider beverages with added electrolytes or consume electrolyte-rich foods to restore balance.

7. Balanced Approach: Individualized Ratios: Experiment with different ratios of protein to carbohydrates based on individual preferences, tolerances, and goals.

Varied Nutrient Sources: Consume a variety of nutrient sources to ensure a well-rounded intake of essential nutrients.

8. Monitoring and adjustments: Listen to your body: Pay attention to how your body responds to different post workout nutrition strategies. Adjust your approach based on individual needs and preferences.

9. Consider Preferences: Tailor post workout nutrition to align with personal taste preferences, ensuring that the chosen foods or beverages are enjoyable and sustainable.

10. Reassess Periodically: As fitness goals, training intensity, or dietary preferences evolve, periodically reassess and adjust your post workout nutrition strategy accordingly.

Integration of Post-Workout Nutrition into Fitness Routines:

Preplanning Meals: Preworkout Nutrition: Consider incorporating elements of post workout nutrition into preworkout meals, ensuring that the body has the necessary nutrients available for both energy during exercise and recovery afterward.

- Balanced Day of Eating: Rather than focusing solely on post workout nutrition, aim for balanced meals throughout the day, distributing macronutrients and micronutrients consistently.

- Education and Awareness: Stay informed about the nutritional needs specific to your fitness goals, ensuring that your post workout nutrition aligns with your objectives.

- Awareness of Individual Responses: Pay attention to how your body responds to different foods and nutrients, adjusting your post workout nutrition based on individual reactions.

- Holistic Approach: Supplements as Supplements: While supplements can be convenient, prioritize whole foods as the foundation of post workout nutrition. Supplements should complement, not replace, a well-rounded diet.

- Incorporate Other Recovery Practices: Combine post workout nutrition with other recovery strategies, such as adequate sleep, hydration, and stress management, for a comprehensive approach to wellbeing.

- Flexibility and adaptability: Variability in Nutrient Ratios: Recognize that the ideal nutrient ratio can vary among individuals and may depend on factors such as workout intensity, duration, and personal preferences.

- Adjustments Based on Training Cycles: Consider adjusting your post workout nutrition strategy based on different training cycles, such as periods of increased intensity or focused training blocks.

Conclusion:

Post workout nutrition is a crucial element in optimizing the benefits of physical activity, supporting recovery, and enhancing overall fitness goals. The combination of protein, carbohydrates, hydration, and other essential nutrients contributes to muscle repair, glycogen replenishment, and reduced exercise-induced stress. Recognizing the individualized nature of post workout nutrition allows individuals to tailor their approach to align with personal preferences, dietary choices, and specific fitness objectives. By integrating effective post workout nutrition strategies into a holistic fitness routine, individual can maximize their efforts, promote sustainable progress, and contribute to long-term wellbeing.

Functional Fitness for Daily Life

Empowering Everyday Movement: The Essence of Functional Fitness

Functional fitness focuses on enhancing the body's ability to perform daily activities efficiently and safely. It goes beyond traditional exercises by incorporating movements that mimic real-life situations. In this exploration, we'll delve into the integration of functional movements and the importance of building core strength for a well-rounded approach to functional fitness.

Integrating Functional Movements: Functional movements are exercises that train the body for activities performed in daily life. These movements engage multiple muscle groups, improve coordination, and enhance the body's overall functionality. By integrating functional movements into a fitness routine, individuals can improve their ability to perform everyday tasks and reduce the risk of injuries related to daily activities.

Examples of Functional Movements:

Squatting: Daily Application: By mimicking the motion of sitting down and standing up, squats strengthen the muscles used in activities like getting in and out of a chair.

Lunging: Daily Application: Walking and going up or down stairs involve lunging-type movements. Incorporating lunges into workouts helps strengthen the muscles involved in these actions.

Pushing and pulling: Daily Application: Pushing a door open, pulling a heavy object or even carrying groceries involves upper body pushing and pulling. Exercises like push-ups and rows target these movements.

Twisting and rotating: Daily Application: Turning to look behind you, reaching for items, or any rotational movement engages the core. Including exercises like Russian twists or wood chops can improve rotational strength.

Carrying: Daily Application: Carrying groceries, lifting a child, or moving household items require strength and stability. Farmers' walks or loaded carries replicate these functional activities.

Benefits of Integrating Functional Movements:

Improved Daily Functionality: Efficient Movement: Functional movements enhance the body's ability to move efficiently in various planes of motion, translating to improved daily functionality.

Joint Mobility: These movements promote joint mobility and flexibility, reducing stiffness and improving the range of motion required for daily activities.

Reduced injury risk: Muscle Symmetry: By engaging multiple muscle groups simultaneously, functional movements contribute to muscle symmetry, reducing the risk of imbalances that can lead to injuries.

Joint Stability: Training functional movements enhances joint stability, protecting against injuries that may arise from unstable joints during everyday activities.

Enhanced Balance and Coordination: Neuromuscular Coordination: Functional movements require the integration of muscles and the nervous system, improving neuromuscular coordination.

Balance Improvement: Incorporating movements that challenge balance and proprioception contributes to improved overall balance.

Time Efficient Workouts: Full-body Engagement: Functional movements often engage multiple muscle groups simultaneously, making workouts more efficient by targeting various areas in one exercise.

Real-Life Application: The efficiency of functional movements' lies in their real-life application, ensuring that the time spent exercising directly translates to improved daily activities.

Incorporating Functional Movements into a Fitness Routine:

Bodyweight Exercises: Squats and Lunges: Incorporate bodyweight squats and lunges to improve lower body strength and mimic movements like sitting and walking.

Pushups and Pull-ups: These exercises engage the upper body in pushing and pulling motions, resembling activities such as pushing doors or pulling objects.

Functional training equipment: Kettle bells and Dumbbells: Implement kettle bell swings and dumbbell movements to add resistance and challenge various muscle groups simultaneously.

Medicine Balls: Use medicine ball exercises for dynamic movements, such as rotational throws and overhead slams, to improve core strength and overall coordination.

MultiPlanar Movements: Rotational Exercises: Include exercises that involve twisting and rotating, such as wood chops or medicine ball twists, to target the core and enhance rotational strength.

Crawling Patterns: Incorporate crawling patterns to engage the entire body, improve coordination, and challenge different muscle groups.

Functional Circuit Training: Circuit Workouts: Design circuit workouts that incorporate a variety of functional movements to keep the routine dynamic and engaging.

Real-Life Scenarios: Structure workouts to mimic real-life scenarios, such as combining lifting movements with walking or carrying exercises.

Progressive Overload: Gradual Progression: Gradually increase the intensity and complexity of functional movements to provide a progressive overload, promoting strength and skill development.

Adaptation to Daily Tasks: Ensure that the functional movements chosen align with the specific daily tasks an individual wants to improve.

Building Core Strength

Core strength is central to overall functional fitness, serving as the foundation for virtually every movement. The core encompasses not only the abdominal muscles but also the muscles of the lower back, pelvis, and hips. A strong core provides stability, balance, and power, influencing posture and the ability to perform daily activities with efficiency and reduced risk of injury.

Importance of Core Strength:

Stabilization and Balance: Spinal Support: The core muscles, including the deep muscles of the spine, provide essential support to the spine, contributing to better posture and reduced strain on the lower back.

Balance Enhancement: A strong core enhances balance, which is crucial for activities like walking, running, and navigating uneven surfaces.

Functional Movement Efficiency: Transfer of Power: Many functional movements involve the transfer of power from the lower body through the core to the upper body. A strong core ensures efficient power transfer.

Improved Coordination: Core strength enhances coordination, allowing for smoother and more controlled movements during daily activities.

Injury Prevention: Reduced Lower Back Strain: Weak core muscles can lead to increased stress on the lower back, potentially resulting in chronic pain. Core strength helps reduce this strain.

Joint Protection: Adequate core strength stabilizes the pelvis and hips, protecting the joints from misalignment and reducing the risk of injuries.

Enhanced Performance in Sports and Activities: Sport-Specific Movements: Many sports and recreational activities require strong core engagement for optimal performance. Building core strength can improve athletic prowess.

Efficient Movement Patterns: Core strength contributes to efficient movement patterns, allowing individuals to excel in activities that demand agility, speed, and coordination.

Effective Core Strengthening Exercises:

Plank Variations: Front Plank: Engages the entire core, including the abdominal muscles, lower back, and stabilizing muscles.

Side Plank: Targets the oblique and lateral core muscles, promoting lateral stability.

Plank with Leg Raises: Incorporates dynamic movement to engage the lower abdominal muscles.

Rotational Exercises: Russian Twists: Targets the obliques and improves rotational strength, which is crucial for functional movements.

Medicine Ball Rotational Throws: This involves twisting and throwing a medicine ball to engage the core muscles dynamically.

Cable Wood Chops utilizes cable machines to simulate wood chopping motions, challenging the core in various planes.

Leg Raises and Flutter Kicks Leg Raises: Targets the lower abdominal muscles and hip flexors, contributing to overall core strength.

Flutter kicks engage the lower abdominal muscles and improve coordination between the lower and upper bodies.

Hollow Body Holds: Full Hollow Body Hold: Challenges the entire core by maintaining a hollow body position, improving overall stability.

Hollow Body Rocking: Adds a dynamic component to the hollow body position, enhancing control and endurance.

Dead Bug Exercise: Opposite Arm and Leg Extensions: This involves extending opposite arms and legs while maintaining a stable core position, improving coordination and stability.

Rotational Dead Bug: introduces a rotational component to the dead bug exercise, engaging the core in multiple directions.

Bridges and hip thrusts: Glute Bridges: Targets the muscles of the glutes, lower back, and core, promoting hip stability.

Barbell Hip Thrusts: Adds resistance to hip thrusts, further challenging the core and glute muscles.

Pilates and yoga movements: Pilates roll-ups focus on controlled movements to strengthen the entire core, particularly the abdominal muscles.

Boat Pose (Navasana): engages the entire core and hip flexors, promoting both strength and balance.

Incorporating Core Exercises into a Fitness Routine:

1. Consistent Integration: Regular Core Workouts: Dedicate specific workout sessions to core exercises, ensuring consistent and targeted training.

2. Incorporate into full body workouts: Integrate core exercises into full body workouts to address the core's role in overall functional fitness.

3. Progressive Overload: Gradual Intensity Increase: Progressively increase the intensity and difficulty of core exercises to provide a challenge and promote strength development.

4. Add Resistance: Introduce resistance gradually, such as holding weights during specific core exercises, to further enhance strength gains.

5. Variety in Movement Patterns: MultiPlanar Exercises: Include core exercises that involve movements in different planes, addressing the core's role in various daily activities.

6. Dynamic vs. Static Movements: Combine dynamic movements (e.g., Russian twists) with static holds (e.g., planks) to target different aspects of core strength.

7. Functional Integration: Functional Movements: Integrate core engagement into functional movements, ensuring that the core is activated during exercises that mimic daily activities.

8. Sport-Specific Training: Tailor core exercises to complement the demands of specific sports or activities an individual enjoys.

9. Balance Training: Incorporate Stability Exercises: Exercises that challenge balance, such as single-leg exercises, inherently engage the core for stability.

10. Bosu Ball Exercises Utilize stability tools like Bosu balls to add an element of instability, requiring increased core activation.

11. Mindful Engagement: Conscious Muscle Engagement: Focus on consciously engaging the core muscles during exercises to maximize their activation.

12. Breathing Awareness: Pay attention to breathing patterns, coordinating breath with movements to enhance core stability.

Real-Life Application of Functional Fitness:

1. Lifting and Carrying:
Lifting Groceries: Functional movements like deadlifts and squats improve the ability to lift and carry heavy objects, such as groceries or household items.

Carrying Children: Core strength is crucial for stability while carrying a child or playing with them on the ground.

2. Daily Mobility:

Bending and Reaching: Functional exercises enhance flexibility and mobility, making daily tasks like bending, reaching, and twisting more manageable.

Getting Up from a Chair: Improved leg and core strength from functional movements assist in getting up from a seated position.

3. Outdoor Activities:

Hiking and Trail Walking: Enhanced balance and coordination from functional fitness contribute to a more enjoyable experience during outdoor activities.

Gardening: Squatting, lifting, and reaching motions, improved by functional movements, make gardening more accessible.

4. Sports Performance:

Improved Golf Swing: Core strength enhances rotational movements, benefiting sports like golf by improving the efficiency and power of the swing.

Running endurance: Functional fitness, including core exercises, supports better posture and endurance while running or participating in cardiovascular activities.

Adapting Functional Fitness to Individual Needs:

5. Assessment of Daily Activities:

Identify Movement Patterns: Assess daily activities to identify common movement patterns, such as lifting, bending, reaching, and twisting.

Tailor Workouts: Tailor functional fitness workouts to address specific movement patterns relevant to an individual's lifestyle and needs.

6.   Individualized Progression:
Start at a Comfortable Level: Begin with functional movements at a comfortable intensity, gradually progressing as strength and confidence increase.

Address Weaknesses: Identify and focus on weaknesses or limitations, addressing them through targeted functional exercises.

7.   Professional Guidance:
Consultation with a Trainer: Seek guidance from a fitness professional or personal trainer to ensure that functional fitness routines align with individual goals and any existing health considerations.

Physical Therapist Support: Individuals with specific health concerns or previous injuries may benefit from guidance and exercises prescribed by a physical therapist.

Conclusion:

Functional fitness serves as a bridge between structured exercise routines and the demands of everyday life. By integrating functional movements and building core strength, individuals enhance their ability to perform daily activities with efficiency, reduce the risk of injury, and increase their overall wellbeing. The practicality of functional fitness lies in its real-life application, making it a valuable approach for individuals seeking to improve not only their physical fitness but also their quality of life. Whether lifting groceries, playing with children, or participating in sports, the benefits of functional fitness extend beyond the gym, enriching the experiences of daily living.

Group Fitness Dynamics

Energizing Together: The Power of Group Fitness

Group fitness has emerged as a popular and effective way for individuals to engage in structured exercise within a communal setting. The synergy of working out together brings a unique dynamic to fitness routines, fostering motivation, camaraderie, and a sense of shared achievement. In this exploration, we'll delve into the benefits of group workouts and highlight some popular group fitness classes that cater to diverse preferences and fitness levels.

The Collective Thrive: Unlocking the Advantages of Group Fitness

Engaging in group workouts extends beyond the physical exertion of exercise. The collective energy, shared goals, and supportive environment create a dynamic that offers numerous benefits for individuals seeking a holistic fitness experience.

Motivation and Accountability:

Group Momentum: The energy of a group workout can be contagious, motivating individuals to push beyond their perceived limits.

Social Accountability: Knowing that others are expecting your presence in the group fosters a sense of accountability, reducing the likelihood of skipping workouts.

Encouragement and Support: Group members often encourage and support each other, creating a positive atmosphere that contributes to individual and collective success.

Variety and Structured Workouts:
Diverse Programming: Group fitness classes offer diverse workout routines, incorporating various exercises and training modalities to keep workouts interesting and challenging.

Expert Guidance: Classes are often led by certified instructors who design structured workouts, ensuring that participants engage in a well-rounded and effective session.

Adaptability: Different classes cater to various fitness levels and preferences, allowing participants to choose sessions that align with their goals and capabilities.

Social Connection and Community:

Build Friendships: Group workouts provide an opportunity to meet likeminded individuals, fostering friendships based on shared fitness goals and experiences.

Sense of Belonging: Being part of a fitness community enhances a sense of belonging, contributing to a positive and supportive environment.

Shared Achievements: Celebrating milestones and achievements together creates a bond among participants, making the fitness journey more enjoyable.

Increased Consistency:
Scheduled Sessions: Group classes often follow a fixed schedule, making it easier for individuals to incorporate regular exercise into their routine.

Routine Establishment: Attending classes at consistent times helps establish a fitness routine, leading to greater adherence and long-term consistency.

Reduced Procrastination: The social and time bound nature of group workouts reduces procrastination, making it less likely for participants to postpone or skip sessions.

Enhanced Performance and Effort:
Competition and Cooperation: The group setting introduces elements of friendly competition and cooperation, motivating individuals to perform at their best.

Pushing Limits: Seeing others work hard can inspire participants to push their own limits, leading to improved performance and fitness gains.

Collective Energy Boost: The energy generated by a group can elevate individual effort, creating an environment where participants challenge themselves more than they might in a solo workout.

Mental Health Benefits:
Stress Reduction: Group workouts offer a social outlet and a break from daily stressors, contributing to improved mental wellbeing.

Positive Environment: The camaraderie and support within a group can create a positive and uplifting atmosphere, reducing feelings of isolation.

Mood Enhancement: Physical activity, combined with the social aspects of group workouts, releases endorphins, leading to improved mood and reduced feelings of anxiety or depression.

Skill Development:
Guidance from Instructors: Instructors in group fitness classes provide guidance on proper form and technique, facilitating skill development.

Learning from Peers: Observing and learning from fellow participants can enhance skill acquisition, especially in activities that involve specific movements or coordination.

Continuous Progression: Regular participation in group classes allows individuals to progress in terms of fitness levels, skill acquisition, and overall performance.

Time Efficiency:
Structured Sessions: Group workouts typically follow a structured format, maximizing the effectiveness of the session within a defined timeframe.

Eliminating Decision Fatigue: Participants don't need to plan their own workouts, reducing decision fatigue and making it simpler to engage in regular exercise.

Optimized Work-to-Rest Ratios: Instructors design workouts with optimized work-to-rest ratios, ensuring that participants make the most of their time in the class.

Popular Group Fitness Classes

From High Intensity to Mindful Movements: A Glimpse into Group Fitness Variety
Group fitness classes encompass a wide range of options, catering to diverse preferences and fitness goals. Whether seeking high-intensity workouts, mindful movements, or dance-based sessions, there's a group fitness class to suit virtually every taste.

High-Intensity Interval Training (HIIT):
Dynamic Workouts: HIIT classes involve alternating between short bursts of intense exercise and periods of rest or lower-intensity activity.

Calorie Burn: HIIT is known for its calorie-burning potential and effectiveness in improving cardiovascular fitness.

Adaptability: HIIT classes can be adapted for various fitness levels, making them suitable for beginners to advanced participants.

Yoga and Pilates:
Mind-Body Connection: Yoga and Pilates classes focus on the integration of breath, movement, and mindfulness.

Flexibility and strength: These classes improve flexibility, core strength, and overall body awareness.

Variety: Different styles of yoga, such as Vinyasa or Hatha, offer varying intensities and approaches to suit individual preferences.

Cycling/Spinning:
Cardiovascular Endurance: Cycling classes provide a high-intensity cardiovascular workout, enhancing endurance and leg strength.

Motivating Atmosphere: The music-driven and instructor-led nature of spinning classes creates a motivating atmosphere for participants.

Adjustable Resistance: Participants can control the resistance on their bikes, allowing for individualized intensity levels.

Dance Fitness:

Energetic Routines: Dance fitness classes, such as Zumba or Dance Cardio, combine dance movements with aerobic exercise.

Fun and Social: Dance fitness is not only a great workout but also a fun and social way to stay active.

Full-body Engagement: Dance routines often engage various muscle groups, providing a full-body workout.

Boot camp Classes:
Total Body Conditioning: Boot camp classes typically incorporate a mix of strength training, cardio, and functional movements.

Team Dynamics: Participants often work in teams or pairs, fostering a sense of camaraderie and teamwork.

Varied Exercises: Bootcamp workouts vary each session, preventing monotony and keeping participants engaged.

Functional Training:
Real-Life Movements: Functional training classes focus on movements that mimic real-life activities, improving overall functionality.

Strength and Mobility: These classes often incorporate strength training and mobility exercises for a well-rounded approach.

Adaptable for All Levels: Functional training classes can be adapted to accommodate participants of varying fitness levels, making them accessible to beginners and challenging for those seeking advanced workouts.

Strength Training Circuits:
Targeted Muscle Work: Strength training circuit classes involve rotating through different exercises targeting specific muscle groups.

Building Lean Muscle: Regular participation can contribute to building lean muscle mass and improving overall strength.

Efficient Workouts: Circuit style training optimizes time, allowing participants to engage in a variety of strength exercises in a single session.

Mindfulness and Meditation Classes:
Stress Reduction: Classes focusing on mindfulness and meditation offer a break from intense physical activity, promoting relaxation and stress reduction.

BodyMind Connection: These sessions often emphasize the connection between the body and mind, fostering mental wellbeing.

Breath Awareness: Mindful movement classes often incorporate breath awareness, contributing to a sense of calm and centering.

Aqua Aerobics:
Low-Impact Exercise: Aqua aerobics classes take place in water, providing a low-impact yet effective workout.

Joint-Friendly: The buoyancy of water reduces impact on joints, making aqua aerobics suitable for individuals with joint concerns.

Full-body Engagement: Water resistance challenges various muscle groups, offering a full-body workout.

Cross Fit Classes:
Functional Fitness Emphasis: Cross Fit is known for its emphasis on functional movements and varied workouts.

Community Spirit: Cross Fit gyms often foster a strong sense of community, with participants encouraging and supporting each other.

WODs (Workouts of the Day): The daily variety of workouts keeps participants engaged and challenged.

Barre Classes:
Ballet-Inspired Workouts: Barre classes draw inspiration from ballet movements, incorporating elements of dance into fitness routines.

Muscle Endurance: Barre workouts focus on small, repetitive movements, promoting muscle endurance and toning.

Core Engagement: Many barre exercises engage the core, contributing to improved stability and posture.

Tai Chi and Qi Gong:
Mindful Movements: Tai Chi and Qi Gong classes involve slow and deliberate movements, promoting mindfulness and relaxation.

Balance and Flexibility: These practices emphasize balance, coordination, and flexibility, making them suitable for all age groups.

Stress Reduction: The meditative nature of Tai Chi and Qi Gong contributes to stress reduction and overall mental wellbeing.

Choosing the Right Group Fitness Class:

Personal Goals:
Fitness Objectives: Consider your fitness goals, whether they involve cardiovascular health, strength building, flexibility, or stress reduction.

Skill Development: Some classes, like dance fitness or martial arts-inspired sessions, offer opportunities for skill development in addition to physical fitness.

Fitness Level:
Entry Level vs. Advanced: Choose a class that aligns with your current fitness level. Many group classes provide modifications to accommodate participants of varying abilities.

Progression: Some classes, such as strength training circuits or CrossFit, can be adapted for progression as your fitness improves.

Personal Preferences:
Enjoyable Activities: Opt for classes that involve activities you enjoy. Whether it's dancing, lifting weights, or practicing mindfulness, selecting enjoyable activities increases adherence.

Social Element: Consider whether you prefer the social dynamic of group classes or if you prefer solo workouts.

Health Considerations:
Joint Health: If you have joint concerns, low-impact classes like aqua aerobics or mindfulness practices might be more suitable.

Medical Clearance: If you have any medical conditions or concerns, consult with a healthcare professional before starting a new fitness regimen.

Variety in Workouts:
Routine Preferences: Decide whether you enjoy routines or prefer varied workouts. Classes like Cross Fit or boot camp offer daily variety, while others may follow a more structured routine.

Combining Classes: Some individuals enjoy a mix of classes throughout the week to ensure a diverse and comprehensive fitness routine.

Conclusion:

Group fitness classes offer a vibrant and diverse landscape for individuals seeking engaging, effective, and enjoyable workouts. The benefits extend beyond physical fitness, encompassing social connections, motivation, and a sense of community. Whether you're drawn to the intensity of high-intensity interval training, the mindfulness of yoga, or the rhythm of dance fitness, there's a group fitness class tailored to your preferences and goals. Exploring different classes allows individuals to discover what resonates with them, making the fitness journey not just a means to an end but an ongoing and fulfilling part of a healthy lifestyle.

Fitness Technology Advancements

From Wearable to Apps: Unveiling the Tech-Infused Fitness Landscape

In recent years, fitness technology has undergone a revolution, transforming the way individuals approach and engage in their fitness journeys. This evolution encompasses a spectrum of innovations, with wearable fitness trackers and workout planning apps standing out as key contributors to this digital fitness era.

Wearable Fitness Trackers

Beyond Counting Steps: The Multifaceted World of Wearable Fitness Technology, Wearable fitness trackers have become ubiquitous accessories, adorning wrists and providing users with a wealth of data to monitor and optimize their fitness endeavors.

1. Step Counters and Activity Tracking:
   Daily Movement Awareness: Wearable trackers, equipped with accelerometers, provide real-time data on steps taken, distance covered, and calories burned throughout the day.

Activity Recognition: Many trackers can automatically identify different activities, from walking and running to cycling and swimming, offering tailored insights for each.

Motivational Element: Visualizing daily activity levels encourages users to meet or exceed their step goals, fostering an active lifestyle.

Heart rate monitoring:
Cardiovascular Insights: Wearables with heart rate monitors enable continuous tracking of heart rate during both rest and exercise.

Efficient Workouts: Users can optimize workout intensity by staying within target heart rate zones, enhancing the efficiency of cardiovascular training.

Recovery Monitoring: Tracking heart rate variability provides insights into the body's recovery status, guiding decisions on rest or more intense workouts.

Sleep Tracking:
Sleep Quality Assessment: Wearables equipped with sleep tracking features analyze sleep patterns, providing insights into the duration and quality of sleep.

Recovery Optimization: Understanding sleep cycles aids in optimizing recovery by influencing factors such as workout timing and intensity.

Sleep Hygiene Improvement: Users receive recommendations for improving sleep hygiene based on tracked data, promoting better sleep habits.

4. Caloric Expenditure Estimation:
Comprehensive Energy Insights: Wearables estimate daily caloric expenditure, combining data on activity levels, heart rate, and basal metabolic rate.

Nutritional Planning: Users can integrate caloric expenditure data with nutritional goals, supporting informed dietary choices.

Weight Management Support: Combining activity and nutrition data aids individuals in achieving weight management goals, whether it's weight loss, maintenance, or muscle gain.

GPS and location tracking:
Outdoor Activity Precision: Integrated GPS allows for accurate tracking of outdoor activities like running, cycling, or hiking.

Route Mapping: Users can review and analyze their exercise routes, identifying areas for improvement or exploring new paths.

Performance Comparison: GPS data facilitates performance analysis by comparing current and past workout metrics on specific routes.

Biometric Measurements:

Advanced Health Metrics: Some wearables offer additional biometric measurements, such as skin temperature, blood oxygen levels, and stress levels.

Holistic Health Insights: Combined biometric data provides a more comprehensive view of overall health, enabling proactive health management.

Early Warning Signs: Deviations from baseline biometric values can serve as early indicators of potential health issues, prompting timely intervention.

Smart watch Integration:
Multifunctional Devices: Many fitness trackers have evolved into smartwatches, offering additional features like call notifications, messaging, and app integration.

Seamless Connectivity: Users can access fitness data, messages, and even control music directly from their wrist, enhancing the overall user experience.

Fitness App Integration: Smartwatches often sync with popular fitness apps, providing a centralized platform for comprehensive health and fitness management.

Community and Social Features:
Social Motivation: Wearables often include features that allow users to connect with friends or a community, fostering friendly competition and support.

Activity Challenges: Users can participate in challenges, set group goals, and share achievements, creating a sense of camaraderie and motivation.

Accountability and Encouragement: Social features provide accountability and encouragement, turning fitness into a shared and enjoyable experience.

Accuracy Concerns:
Variable Accuracy: The accuracy of wearables can vary based on factors such as device quality, placement, and individual differences.

Heart Rate Variability: Accuracy in measuring heart rate during intense workouts or high-intensity intervals may be challenging for certain devices.

Battery Life and Charging:
Frequent Charging: Depending on usage and features, wearables may require frequent charging, potentially interrupting continuous tracking.

Long-Term Battery Durability: Over time, the battery life of wearables may degrade, impacting the device's overall longevity.

Data Security and Privacy:
Sensitivity of Health Data: Wearables collect sensitive health data, raising concerns about data security and privacy.

Data Sharing Policies: Users should be aware of how their health data is stored, shared, and used by wearable manufacturers or associated apps.

Compatibility with Devices:
Interoperability Problems: Different cellphones and operating systems may not be compatible with one another, which might restrict certain features or functions.

Syncing Challenges: When attempting to transmit data from wearables to companion applications, users may run into syncing challenges that affect the smooth integration of fitness data.

Goals for the Future:

Healthcare Integration:
Health Monitoring Partnerships: Manufacturers of wearables and healthcare providers are creating partnerships as wearable technology is further incorporated into healthcare efforts.

Remote Patient Monitoring: Wearable technology has the potential to provide remote patient monitoring, giving medical personnel access to track vital signs and other health parameters from a distance.

Health Insights for Physicians: Wearable data may provide insightful information to medical professionals, facilitating more individualized and data-driven treatment.

Technological Developments in Sensors:

Miniaturization and Precision: As sensor technology continues to progress, it is anticipated that a wider variety of health measurements will be captured by more accurate and smaller sensors.

Continuous Monitoring: Wearables in the future could provide continuous vital sign monitoring, allowing for real-time health evaluations.

Biochemical tracking: As wearable technology advances, it may become possible to integrate biochemical sensors into certain models. This would enable the tracking of particular biomarkers in the body and provide even more detailed health data.

Integration of Artificial Intelligence:
Data Analysis and Personalization: By incorporating artificial intelligence (AI), fitness data analysis will be improved, yielding more individualized conclusions and suggestions.

Predictive Health Modeling: Wearables using AI algorithms may be able to forecast health trends and notify users and medical professionals of any problems before they materialize.

Adaptive Coaching: Based on user performance, objectives, and fluctuating fitness levels, AI-driven coaching features might modify exercise regimens in real time.

Improved user experience:
Improved User Interfaces: Future wearables could have streamlined, user-friendly interfaces with enhanced functionality.

Augmented Reality (AR): Using AR in conjunction with other technologies might improve the user experience by offering real-time training coaching and immersive fitness experiences.

Voice and Gesture Control: Advanced control features like voice commands or gesture recognition may be included in wearables to provide more convenient engagement while exercising.

Applications for Scheduling and Tracking Exercises

Moving Beyond Pen and Paper: The Digital Era of Exercise Scheduling

Apps for planning and tracking workouts have become more popular with wearable fitness trackers, giving consumers the unparalleled ease of organizing their fitness regimens and tracking their progress.

Tailored Exercise Schedules:
Tailored Fitness Regimens: Apps enable users to design or adhere to customized exercise schedules that take into account their fitness level, objectives, and preferred forms of exercise.

Variety and Progression: A wide variety of exercise regimens, from cardio and strength training to flexibility and mindfulness activities, are available to users.

Adaptive Planning: Certain applications modify training regimens in response to user input, changing the level of difficulty and the exercises chosen to correspond with each user's progress.

In-the-moment exercise advice:
Form Corrections: Apps often include form advice and video demonstrations to walk users through exercises to make sure they are doing them correctly.

Audio Cues: To improve the whole training experience, applications may include audio cues for timing repetitions, intervals, or rest times throughout workouts.

Visual Timers: Devices with visual timers may help users stay on top of exercise durations and intervals.

Analytics and Progress Monitoring:
Performance Metrics: Users of workout applications may monitor parameters including repetitions, sets, weight lifted, and times to completion.

Graphical Representations: Charts and graphs that show development over time provide a clear summary of the advancements that have been made.

Goal Achievement: Using the app, users may create personalized fitness objectives, monitor their progress toward benchmarks, and acknowledge successes.

Wearables Integration:
Data Syncing: A lot of fitness applications easily connect to wearable fitness trackers, combining data into an all-encompassing picture.

Holistic Health Monitoring: Users may monitor their overall fitness and health, including exercise and activity details, by combining data from wearables and apps.

Automatic Workout Logging: The app's workout logs may automatically include wearable data, such as heart rate and steps, to expedite the monitoring process.

Nutritional Monitoring and Counseling:
> Meal Logging: A few fitness applications provide tools for keeping track of daily nutrition, enabling users to keep an eye on their intake of calories and distribution of macronutrients.

Nutritional advice: To encourage a holistic approach to health, apps may provide users with meal planning and nutritional advice depending on their exercise objectives.

Integration with Diet Applications: The management of fitness-related factors is improved when there is integration with specialized diet and nutrition applications, guaranteeing a well-rounded approach to wellbeing.

Social and Community Aspects:
Workout Sharing: Within the app's community or on social media, users may post updates about their progress, accomplishments, and finished workouts.

Peer Support: Through social features, users may interact with peers and exchange fitness advice as well as words of encouragement and support.

Competition and Challenges: Workout applications often include challenges and contests, encouraging users to share mutually beneficial rivalries and common objectives.

Integrating AI and Virtual Coaching:
Virtual Coaches: A few applications make use of virtual coaching capabilities to provide users with advice and comments in real time while working out.

AI-Driven Suggestions: Based on user data analysis, artificial intelligence may provide tailored exercise suggestions and modify programs in response to individual progress.

Feedback Loops: Apps have the option to include feedback loops, which collect user feedback on training experiences in order to improve coaching algorithms over time.

Inclusivity and Accessibility:
Adaptable workouts: A lot of fitness applications provide adaptable workouts to suit people with different degrees of fitness, skills, and preferences.

Inclusive Programming: By addressing a variety of requirements, inclusive exercise programming increases accessibility to fitness for people from a variety of backgrounds and situations.

Customizable exercises: Users may often alter exercises to fit their needs in terms of equipment, time, or personal preferences.

Overload in App Selection:

Overwhelming Choices: With so many fitness applications available, users may get overwhelmed with options and find it difficult to decide which one best suits their requirements.

Suscription Costs: Certain in-app customized plans or sophisticated features may have a subscription fee, which affects financial planning.

Adherence by Users:
Consistency Challenges: Although applications make life easier, maintaining user adherence to exercise regimens is still a problem for certain people.

Motivating strategies: To promote sustained engagement, apps must have powerful motivating techniques, including goal setting tools, progress monitoring, and reminders.

Privacy Issues with Data:
Sensitive Information: Because fitness applications gather private and health-related data, strong privacy safeguards are required to protect user data.

Data Sharing Practices: To ensure transparency and consent, users should be informed about how their data is shared, kept, and utilized.

Interoperability and Sync:
Device Compatibility: The smooth integration of fitness data may be impacted by an app's restricted compatibility with certain hardware or operating systems.

Syncing Issues: Users may have issues with syncing, which might compromise the precision of progress tracking and exercise data.

Goals for the Future:

Integration of Virtual Reality (VR):
Immersion Workouts: VR integration in fitness applications in the future might provide users with immersive fitness experiences that mimic different training settings or surroundings.

Interactive Training Sessions: Virtual reality has the potential to provide interactive training sessions, whereby users may interact with virtual teachers or partake in gamified exercises.

Enhanced Motivation: By producing dynamic and captivating training settings, virtual reality's immersive quality may improve motivation.

Integrated Biometric Feedback:
Real-Time Biometrics: With advancements, wearable sensor integration may become possible for applications, allowing for real-time biometric feedback during exercise.

Adaptive Coaching: Based on the user's current physiological condition, apps may use continuous biometric data to modify coaching levels and instructions.

Biofeedback Training: By using biofeedback strategies, users may be able to maximize their training results and control their stress levels.

Personalized machine learning:
Dynamic exercise programs: Based on user data analysis, machine learning algorithms may modify exercise programs dynamically to maintain their efficacy and relevance over time.

Behavior Prediction: Using machine learning, apps may be able to anticipate user behavior patterns and provide users with motivating material, ideas, and timely reminders that match their fitness regimens.

Individualized suggestions: Taking into account variables like preferences, progress, and past data, machine learning may be able to provide more individualized dietary and activity suggestions.

Augmented Reality for Exercise Program Guidance:
Interactive Exercise Demonstrations: Virtual trainers might assist users through guided exercises using augmented reality (AR), which could bring exercise demonstrations to life.

Real-Time Form Corrections: AR features have the potential to provide real-time form corrections, improving exercise safety and efficacy.

Spatial Awareness: AR may provide users with spatial clues to help them position and move correctly while doing workouts.

Virtual Exercises for Collaboration:
Synchronous Training Sessions: Upcoming applications could make synchronous training possible, enabling users to participate in online group sessions in real time.

Interactive Challenges: Interactive games and challenges may be included in cooperative virtual exercises to promote a feeling of camaraderie and mutual success.

Social Connectivity: To improve the community nature of group exercise, virtual workouts may include social features like voice chat or avatars.

Integrating Biohacking
Data-Driven Optimization: Biohacking concepts may be incorporated into apps, enabling users to monitor and improve a range of health-related factors, including rest, stress, and recuperation.

Biofeedback Training: By using biohacking methods, applications may help users optimize their way of life for maximum effectiveness and wellbeing.

Goal-Specific Strategies: The integration of biohacking techniques may provide users with customized approaches to attaining certain fitness and health objectives.

Result:
 An era when people may use fitness applications and wearables to improve their health and wellbeing has been brought about by the convergence of technology and fitness. With their wide range of functions, wearable fitness trackers have emerged as essential instruments for tracking health indicators, physical activity, and even the quality of sleep. Apps for organizing and tracking workouts have also developed into dynamic platforms that provide

social interaction, progress tracking, and personalized coaching in addition to leading users through exercises.

The difficulties and issues surrounding fitness technology, such as worries about data privacy and accuracy, highlight the need for ongoing development and user education. With wearables and applications ready to connect seamlessly and make use of virtual reality, machine learning, augmented reality, and biohacking to create even more customized and interesting fitness experiences, the future of technology is full of fascinating possibilities.

The fitness industry is expanding because of the marriage of human activity and technological advancement, which provides a wide range of options to suit various tastes, objectives, and lifestyles. The secret to navigating this new frontier of digital fitness for people is to use technology as a helpful ally rather than merely a tool as they pursue holistic health and wellbeing. One stride, one rep, and one digital engagement at a moment, technology is enabling people to take control of their own fitness destiny. This may be achieved via interactive exercise apps or subtle nudges from wearables.

Injury Prevention and Management: Guarding the Temple: An All-Inclusive Manual for Injury Avoidance and Recovery in the Gym. Injury management and prevention are crucial factors to take into account while aiming for fitness. This investigation explores frequent injuries sustained in the gym, their causes, and useful rehabilitation activities to promote a proactive attitude toward health and wellbeing.

Typical Wellness Injuries

Knowing Your Weaknesses: Recognizing and Treating Exercise-Related Injuries

Although the gym is a refuge for many looking to alter their bodies, there are hazards involved, since hard exercise may lead to injury. It's critical to identify frequent gym injuries in order to avoid injuries and provide appropriate care.

Depression and anxiety:
Causes: Sprains (ligament injuries) or strains (muscle or tendon injuries) may result from overexertion, incorrect warmup techniques, or lifting weights above one's capabilities.

Prevention: A sufficient warmup, appropriate form, and a steady increase in intensity all contribute to a lower chance of sprains and strains.

Management: During the early stages of rehabilitation, R.I.C.E. (rest, ice, compression, and elevation) is often advised. This is followed by regulated mobility and strengthening activities.

Tendinitis:
Causes: Repetitive movements or incorrect form may cause overuse of certain tendons, which can lead to tendinitis and inflammation.

Prevention: Changing up your exercises, using the right form, and taking enough time off in between strenuous sessions all help to avoid tendinitis.

Treatment: The treatment strategy may include anti-inflammatory drugs, targeted exercise to strengthen the surrounding muscles, and rest.

Tears in the Ligament:
Causes: Acute impact, poor landing technique, or unnatural weightlifting motions may rupture ligaments, often damaging shoulder and knee joints.

Prevention: Ligament tears may be avoided by emphasizing good form, using the right tools, and including balance and stability exercises.

Management: In extreme situations, surgery could be required. A thorough rehabilitation program would then be implemented to regain strength and mobility.

Injuries from Rotator Cuffs:
Causes: Rotator cuff injuries, which are characterized by discomfort and restricted shoulder mobility, may be brought on by overhead lifting, poor shoulder mechanics, or unexpected trauma.

Prevention: Rotator cuff strengthening exercises, a thorough warmup, and avoiding excessive overhead motions all aid in the prevention of injuries.

Management: A typical rehabilitation strategy involves rotator cuff strengthening, physical therapy, rest, and a gradual return to shoulder activities.

Back Strains:
Causes: Back problems, such as muscular strains or herniated discs, may be caused by improper form while lifting weights, stressing the spine, or making abrupt movements.

Prevention: Exercises that strengthen the core, safe lifting practices, and avoiding prolonged spinal strain all help to prevent back problems.

Management: Recuperation may sometimes be aided by physical therapy or chiropractic adjustments, rest, and specific workouts for the back muscles.

Shin Splints:
Causes: High-impact exercises like running and leaping may cause repetitive stress on the shinbone and the tissues that connect muscles to the bone.

Prevention: Lower-impact workouts, appropriate footwear, and a gradual increase in intensity may all help avoid shin splints.

Management: Common treatments for shin splints include rest, ice, and exercises that target the strength and flexibility of the calves.

Tears in the ACL and MCL in the knee:

Causes: Tears in the anterior cruciate ligament (ACL) or medial collateral ligament (MCL) may occur from abrupt changes in direction, poor landing technique, or direct contact.

Prevention: You may lower your chance of knee injuries by utilizing protective gear, practicing landing technique correction, and strengthening the muscles around your knee.

Management: Depending on the severity, a systematic rehabilitation program may come after rest, physical therapy, or surgery as a form of treatment.

Fractures from stress:
Causes: Stress fractures, which are often seen in weight-bearing bones like the foot or shin, are microscopic fissures in bones caused by overuse, repeated impact, or insufficient rest.

Prevention: Stress fractures may be avoided by including rest days into the exercise program, gradually increasing the intensity, and using appropriate footwear.

Management: Activities that don't place undue strain on the injured bones, in addition to rest, are essential for the healing of stress fractures. It is advisable to gradually resume regular activities.

Overexertion and dehydration:
Causes: Dehydration, lightheadedness, and, in extreme situations, heat-related disorders may result from dehydration and straining the body over its breaking point.

Prevention: The best ways to avoid dehydration and overexertion are to stay hydrated, understand your own limitations, and acclimate to rigorous exercises gradually.

Management: Treating dehydration and overexertion requires prompt rest, fluids, and, in extreme situations, medical intervention.

Tennis or golfer's elbow:
Causes: Elbow tendon irritation and soreness may result from repetitive gripping or wrist motions, which are typical in exercises like weightlifting.

Prevention: Using ergonomic equipment, using proper technique, and including workouts that strengthen the forearms will help avoid these disorders.

Treatment: The treatment strategy includes ice, rest, and activities to strengthen the muscles in the forearm. It is recommended that gripping activities be gradually resumed throughout the healing process.

Exercises for Rehabilitation

The Recovery Process: Specific Exercises for Rehabilitating Injuries

Exercises for rehabilitation are essential to the healing process after an accident. The goal of these exercises is to reduce the chance of rein jury while maximizing strength, flexibility, and functioning.

Exercises to Strengthen Your Rotator Cuff:

Internal and External Rotations: To work on the rotator cuff muscles, do internal and external rotation exercises with light dumbbells or resistance bands.

Scapular Retraction: By pulling and compressing the shoulder blades together, you may strengthen the muscles that run between them.

External Rotation While Lying on Your Side: Lift a small dumbbell away from your body while lying on your side and concentrate on activating your external rotators.

Activities to strengthen your core:
Plank Variations: Include plank exercises, such as side planks and front planks, to work the whole core.

Russian Twists: While gripping a weight or medicine ball, spin your torso while sitting or standing, working your oblique.

Leg Raises: While lying flat on your back, extend your legs upward by using your lower abdominal muscles.

Strengthening Your Hamstrings and Quadriceps
Leg Press: Push against resistance to strengthen the quadriceps by using a leg press machine or resistance bands.

Hamstring Curls: Use a stability ball or a dedicated machine to perform hamstring curls, targeting the muscles at the back of the thigh.

Step-ups: Step onto a platform, engaging both quadriceps and hamstrings as you lift your body.

Glute Activation Exercises:
Bridges: Lie on your back and lift your hips toward the ceiling, engaging the glutes. Progress by adding resistance or performing single-leg bridges.

Clamshells: Sidelying, open and close your legs like a clamshell, targeting the gluteus medius.

Lunges: Perform lunges to engage the glutes and strengthen the muscles around the hips.

Balance and Stability Exercises:
Single-Leg Stance: Stand on one leg, engaging the core and stabilizing muscles. Progress by closing your eyes or adding dynamic movements.

BOSU Ball Exercises: Utilize a BOSU ball for exercises that challenge balance, such as squats or lunges.

Proprioceptive Training: Include exercises that challenge proprioception, like standing on an unstable surface or using balance discs.

Flexibility and Mobility Exercises:

Dynamic Stretching: Incorporate dynamic stretching into warm-up routines, involving controlled, active movements through a full range of motion.

Foam Rolling: Use foam rollers to release tension in muscles and improve flexibility.

Yoga or Pilates: Regular practice of yoga or Pilates can enhance flexibility, mobility, and overall body awareness.

Functional Movement Patterns:
Squat Variations: Perform squats with proper form, focusing on engaging the core and maintaining alignment.

Dead lifts: Execute deadlifts with proper technique, engaging the posterior chain, and promoting functional movement.

Push and Pull Exercises: Incorporate pushing (e.g., bench press) and pulling (e.g., rows) exercises to promote balanced strength.

Cardiovascular Exercise:
Low-Impact Options: Choose low-impact cardiovascular exercises like cycling or swimming during the rehabilitation phase.

Gradual Progression: Progress to higher-impact activities gradually, ensuring the body can tolerate the demands of cardiovascular exercise.

Interval Training: Implement interval training to gradually increase intensity while allowing for adequate recovery.

Neuromuscular Control Exercises:
Plyometric Movements: Controlled plyometric exercises, such as box jumps or lateral jumps, enhance neuromuscular control.

Cone Drills: Perform agility drills using cones or markers to improve coordination and response time.

Mirror Exercises: Use mirrors to perform exercises that involve coordination and symmetrical movements for both sides of the body.

Cross Training Activities:
Swimming: Incorporate swimming for a full-body, low-impact workout that enhances cardiovascular fitness and muscular endurance.

Cycling: Engage in cycling, either outdoors or using stationary bikes, to build leg strength and cardiovascular fitness.

Rowing: Rowing exercises, whether on a rowing machine or in water, provide a low-impact way to strengthen the upper body and core.

Guidelines for Injury Prevention and Rehabilitation:

Consultation with Healthcare Professionals:
Preexisting Conditions: Individuals with preexisting health conditions should consult healthcare professionals before starting a new exercise regimen.

Injury Assessment: In cases of injuries, seek timely assessment and guidance from medical professionals to determine the appropriate course of action.

Gradual Progression:
Avoid overtraining: Gradually increase the intensity, duration, or frequency of workouts to allow the body to adapt and reduce the risk of overtraining.

Listen to the body: Pay attention to signals of fatigue, discomfort, or pain, and adjust the workout accordingly to prevent injuries.

Proper Warm-Up and Cool-Down:
Dynamic Warmup: Incorporate dynamic stretching and movements into the warmup routine to prepare muscles for activity.

Cool Down: Allow time for a cool down phase, including static stretching, to promote flexibility and aid in the recovery process.

Technique and Form:
Educate yourself: Learn and practice proper exercise techniques to ensure correct form during workouts.

Professional Guidance: Seek guidance from fitness professionals or trainers to ensure proper technique, especially when starting a new exercise or lifting routine.

Balanced Training:
Muscle Balance: Design workouts that address muscle imbalances, ensuring balanced strength and flexibility.

Variety in Exercises: Include a variety of exercises to target different muscle groups and movement patterns, reducing the risk of overuse injuries.

Rest and Recovery:
Adequate Rest Days: Schedule regular rest days to allow the body time to recover and prevent overtraining.

Sleep Quality: Prioritize sufficient and quality sleep, as it plays a crucial role in the body's recovery and repair processes.

Nutrition and Hydration:
Balanced Diet: Maintain a balanced diet rich in nutrients to support overall health, including the recovery of muscles and tissues.

Hydration: Stay well hydrated, as proper hydration is essential for joint lubrication, muscle function, and overall wellbeing.

Monitoring Warning Signs:
Persistent Pain: Address persistent pain or discomfort promptly, as it may be indicative of underlying issues that require attention.

Inflammation and Swelling: Monitor for signs of inflammation or swelling after workouts, as these may be indicators of overuse or injury that needs attention.

Range of Motion: Track changes in range of motion, as limitations or discomfort may signify developing issues that need assessment.

Fatigue and Burnout: Be aware of signs of excessive fatigue or burnout, such as chronic tiredness, irritability, or a decline in performance.

Rehabilitation Progression:

Assessment and Diagnosis:
Professional Evaluation: Seek assessment and diagnosis from healthcare professionals, including physicians, physiotherapists, or sports medicine specialists.

Imaging Studies: Depending on the injury, imaging studies like X-rays, MRIs, or ultrasounds may be necessary for a comprehensive diagnosis.

Rest and Initial Recovery:
Immediate Rest: In the initial phase post-injury, prioritize rest to allow the body to begin the healing process.

R.I.C.E.: Employ the R.I.C.E. protocol (Rest, Ice, Compression, and Elevation) as appropriate for managing acute injuries and reducing inflammation.

Professional Guidance:
Physical Therapy: Engage in physical therapy sessions under the guidance of qualified professionals to target specific rehabilitation needs.

Rehabilitation Plan: Work with physical therapists to develop a customized rehabilitation plan that addresses individual strengths, weaknesses, and goals.

Progressive Exercises:
Gradual Introduction: Introduce exercises gradually, starting with low-intensity movements and progressively increasing difficulty.

Monitoring Responses: Pay attention to how the body responds to exercises, adjusting intensity or type based on comfort and progress.

Strength and Stability: Prioritize exercises that enhance both strength and stability, aiming to restore functionality to preinjury levels.

Cardiovascular Conditioning:
Low-Impact Options: Begin with low-impact cardiovascular exercises, gradually increasing intensity as cardiovascular fitness improves.

Interval Training: Implement interval training cautiously, ensuring it aligns with the body's readiness for increased cardiovascular demands.

Monitoring Tolerance: Monitor cardiovascular tolerance and adjust the duration and intensity of workouts accordingly.

Neuromuscular Control:

Coordination Exercises: Incorporate exercises that challenge coordination and neuromuscular control, aiding in the restoration of functional movement patterns.

Proprioceptive Training: Include activities that enhance proprioception, contributing to improved joint stability and awareness.

Balance Progressions: Progress balance exercises from simple to more complexes as stability improves.

Functional Movement Assessment:
Functional Testing: Engage in functional movement assessments to evaluate the readiness to return to specific activities or sports.

Biomechanical Analysis: Consider biomechanical analysis, especially for activities involving repetitive or specialized movements.

Consultation with professionals: For a thorough assessment, get advice from professionals like movement specialists or biomechanics experts.

Steppe back Reentry into Activities:
Incremental Progression: Reintroduce sports or activities gradually, making sure each step is well tolerated and does not cause setbacks.

Performance Monitoring: During the return-to-play period, keep an eye on performance and evaluate any indications of weakness, pain, or altered movement patterns.

Cooperation with Coaches: Work together with trainers or coaches to make sure that the return to routine training or competitive settings goes well.

Psychological Assistance:
Addressing Apprehensions: Through open communication and support, identify and address psychological concerns, such as worries or apprehensions associated with rein jury.

Mental Resilience: Practice mindfulness, positive affirmations, and visualization techniques to strengthen your mental toughness.

Professional Counseling: Should psychological variables have a substantial influence on the recovery process, think about obtaining professional counseling or mental health help.

Impacts and Things to Take into Account in Injury Prevention and Rehabilitation:

Adherence by Patients:
Consistency in Rehabilitation: People may find it difficult to stick with rehabilitation programs and to be consistent over the course of their recovery.

Motivational Strategies: To improve adherence, use motivational techniques, including goal setting, monitoring progress, and providing positive reinforcement.

Separate Variability:

Unique Rehabilitation Needs: Because every person's injuries and recovery process are different, rehabilitation methods must be tailored to each individual.

Tailored Programs: Taking into account the patient's general health, rehabilitation programs need to be designed to target a particular patient's strengths, weaknesses, and limits.

Deciding to Return to Play:
Collaborative Decision-Making: Healthcare providers, coaches, and the player should all work together to make decisions about the player's return to play.

Objective Criteria: Establish objective standards to inform return-to-play choices, such as the outcomes of functional tests and biomechanical evaluations.

Overcoming Obstacles of the Mind:
Anxiety of reinjury: Resolving this anxiety is essential since psychological obstacles may obstruct recovery and confidence in going back to routine activities.

Gradual Exposure: Positive reinforcement combined with gradual exposure to sports and activities may assist people in overcoming psychological obstacles.

Keeping Rest and Intensity in Check:
Striking a Balance: Effective rehabilitation depends on striking the correct balance between exercise intensity and rest periods.

Monitoring exhaustion: Constant observation of one's state of exhaustion helps in avoiding overtraining, which may impede the recuperation process.

Initiatives in Education:
Raising Awareness: Education campaigns need to concentrate on educating people about safe warmup methods, injury prevention tactics, and the value of paying attention to their bodies.

Educating Coaches and Trainers: As they are essential in preventing injuries, coaches and trainers must be knowledgeable about the newest techniques and approaches.

Technology Integration:
Biomechanical Feedback: Using technology in conjunction with biomechanical feedback tools may help avoid injuries and provide insightful information about movement patterns.

Remote Rehabilitation: Programs for remote rehabilitation that are facilitated by technology may improve accessibility and adherence to treatment regimens.

Support for Nutrition:
Nutritional Considerations: Since a healthy diet is crucial to the healing process, including nutritional advice and support is crucial.

Timing of Hydration and Nutrients: Stress the significance of timing nutrients and hydration in accordance with an individual's energy requirements and demands for recuperation.

Next Developments in Injury Avoidance and Rehabilitation:

Biomechanics Advancements:
Real-time biomechanical analysis: With the potential for future advancements, this feature might provide immediate feedback on movement patterns during rehabilitation activities.

Wearable Biomechanics: Wearable technology that can evaluate biomechanics has the potential to become a vital tool for injury prevention and rehabilitation.

Tailored Rehab Programs:
Genetic and Biomarker Insights: Based on each person's unique reaction to exercise, personalized rehabilitation strategies may include genetic and biomarker data.

Artificial Intelligence: In order to identify trends and develop individualized rehabilitation plans, artificial intelligence may be used to analyze massive datasets.

Rehabilitation with Virtual Reality:
Immersive Rehabilitation Settings: People may participate in therapeutic activities in a simulated setting by using virtual reality to create immersive rehabilitation settings.

Motor Imagery Training: Using virtual reality to support motor imagery training might help people improve neuromuscular control and mentally practice motions.

Remote Monitoring and Telemedicine:

Remote Rehabilitation Platforms: The incorporation of telemedicine may facilitate programs for remote rehabilitation, where medical practitioners track patients' progress via online portals.

Wearable Monitoring Devices: As wearable technology advances, it may be possible for it to provide real-time movement data, enabling remote rehabilitation plan evaluation and modification.

Integrating Mind and Body:
Mindfulness-Based Rehabilitation: Stress reduction, mental resilience building, and overall wellbeing promotion are some of the goals that mindfulness practices may help with in rehabilitation programs.

Biofeedback Techniques: In the future, biofeedback methods that enable people to get real-time information on their physiological reactions during rehabilitation could be developed.

Gamification and Exergaming:
Interactive Rehabilitation Games: Rehabilitation exercises may be made more interesting by using exergaming, which is the use of interactive video games that require physical mobility.

Gamified Progress Monitoring: Gamification components might be added to progress monitoring to provide people incentives and prizes for participation and accomplishments.

Networks of Peers and Community Support:

Virtual Support Communities: Social media and online platforms may act as virtual communities where people going through rehabilitation can connect and exchange experiences.

Formalized peer mentoring programs have the potential to link those undergoing recovery with others who have successfully traversed comparable rehabilitation journeys.

Integrated Holistic Wellness:
Nutritional Counseling: Taking into account the influence of food on healing and general wellbeing, rehabilitation programs may include individualized nutritional counseling.

Mental Health Services: By treating psychological issues and guaranteeing a holistic approach to wellbeing, mental health assistance may play a crucial role in rehabilitation.

Preventive Evaluation and Screening:
Pre-rehabilitation assessments: It could become common practice to include screening exams for preventative care before participating in strenuous physical activities.

Early Intervention: By identifying possible vulnerabilities early on, specific treatments may be implemented to lower the risk of injuries before they happen.

Models of Collaborative Care:
Multidisciplinary Teams: Future forms of rehabilitation could include collaborative care, in which experts from different fields collaborate to meet the unique requirements of patients.

Integrated Care Platforms: All-inclusive platforms that include exercise, rehabilitation, and healthcare services may improve coordination and communication amongst various healthcare professionals.

Empowerment and Education:
Digital Education Platforms: A plethora of online educational materials may be available to people, offering knowledge on how to avoid injuries, recover from them, and maintain general health.

Empowerment Through Technology: With tools and resources for self-guided exercise and progress monitoring, technology might enable people to actively participate in their rehabilitation.

Result:

Fitness-related injury prevention and rehabilitation are changing as a result of technological breakthroughs, individualized methods, and attention to overall wellbeing. Future rehabilitation experiences might be more personalized, interesting, and easily accessible by using advancements in telemedicine, virtual reality, biomechanics, and other fields.

The future of injury prevention and rehabilitation is one in which data-driven insights, collaborative care models, and technological integration become essential components. Important elements of this vision include developing a sense of community support, integrating mind-body practices, and customizing rehabilitation regimens to each patient's requirements. Thanks to these developments, the road from injury prevention to rehabilitation is no longer merely a recuperation procedure; rather, it is a life-changing experience that corresponds with the many requirements and goals that people have on their journeys toward optimum health and fitness.

A proactive attitude toward injury prevention, a sophisticated comprehension of rehabilitation, and a comprehensive embrace of wellbeing that goes beyond physical healing are all encouraged by the changing environment. In this future, science, technology, and human resilience will work in unison to transform how we approach and negotiate the complex process of protecting and maintaining the body's temple, making sure it remains strong, adaptable, and prepared for the demands of a full and active life.

Body Fat Loss and Composition

Discovering the Methods for Long-Term Fat Loss and Body Composition

Achieving and maintaining a robust and healthy physique in the context of exercise and wellbeing mostly depends on comprehending body composition and implementing sustainable fat reduction techniques. This investigation explores the complexities of body fat percentage, its importance for general health, and useful tactics for those looking to lose fat in a long-term and sustainable way.

Knowing the Percentage of Body Fat

Going Beyond the Figures: Getting Around the Body Composition Terrain

Body composition, and more especially body fat percentage, is an important measure that extends beyond the narrow perspective of weight control. It offers a sophisticated comprehension of the body's distribution of fat, lean, and other components. A thorough investigation of body fat percentage entails understanding its importance, how it's measured, and the health consequences of varying ranges.

1. Importance of Body Fat Ratio:

Holistic Health Indicator: Taking into account the percentage of body mass that is made up of fat tissue, body fat percentage provides a more thorough evaluation of health than weight alone.

Metabolic Health: Variations in body fat may have an effect on metabolic health, which in turn can affect variables like insulin sensitivity, cholesterol levels, and cardiovascular health in general.

Performance and Functionality: Optimal body fat percentages are often linked to improved performance and functional abilities in athletes and fitness enthusiasts.

2. Methods of Quantification:

Dual-Energy X-ray Absorptiometry (DEXA): DEXA scans provide a very precise way to determine body composition by differentiating between bone density, fat mass, and lean mass.

Bioelectrical Impedance Analysis (BIA): Based on the idea that fat conducts less electricity than muscle, BIA devices detect the resistance of electrical flow through the body to estimate the proportion of body fat.

Skinfold Calipers: Skinfold calipers measure the thickness of the skin at certain body locations to assess the amount of subcutaneous fat.

Hydrostatic Weighing: This technique uses the idea that fat is less dense than lean mass to measure a person's body density by immersing them in water.

Air Displacement Plethysmography (Bod Pod): This noninvasive technique of body composition assessment measures air displacement and is an alternative to hydrostatic weighing.

Infrared Interactance: By measuring how much infrared light is absorbed as it penetrates the skin and underlying tissue, infrared interactance devices calculate the proportion of body fat.

3. The Effects of Body Fat Percentage on Health:
Essential vs. store fat: It's important to understand the distinction between store fat, which is linked to energy

reserves, and essential fat, which is required for physiological processes.

Hormonal Influence: Adipose tissue affects hormones linked to hunger, metabolism, and reproductive processes, and body fat plays a part in this control.

Distribution Patterns: Different body fat distributions, such as visceral fat around organs vs. subcutaneous fat under the skin, may have distinct effects on health outcomes.

Obesity-Related Conditions: Conditions including type 2 diabetes, cardiovascular disease, and several malignancies have been related to high body fat percentages, particularly when these percentages are concentrated around important organs.

Long-Term Fat Loss Techniques

Guiding the Course for Durable Transformation: Empirical Methods for Reducing Body Fat

Reducing body fat sustainably requires a comprehensive strategy that includes food decisions, exercise, and lifestyle adjustments. While extreme methods and fad diets may promise immediate benefits, they often overlook long-term durability. This section looks at evidence-based tactics that put long-term change ahead of quick fixes that won't work.

1. Nutrition in Balance:

Caloric Deficit: In order to achieve sustainable fat reduction, one must usually create a caloric deficit, which is an excess of energy expenditure over calories consumed. This causes the body to burn stored fat for energy.

Macronutrient Distribution: Sustainable fat reduction depends on striking a balance between macronutrients (fats, proteins, and carbs) that promotes general health and satiety.

Whole Foods Emphasis: Giving whole, nutrient-dense foods precedence over processed ones promotes general health by offering vital vitamins, minerals, and fiber.

2. Conscientious Consumption:
Conscious Consumption: To avoid overindulging, mindful eating entails paying attention to what is being eaten, appreciating tastes, and identifying signs of hunger and fullness.

Emotional Eating Awareness: Breaking the pattern of emotional eating requires recognizing the emotions that set off an eating attack as well as creating other coping strategies.

Portion Control: Keeping a balance between calorie intake and expenditure is facilitated by an understanding of proper portion proportions.

3. Continuous physical exercise:

Combination of Cardio and Strength Training: Lean muscle mass is preserved, while total fat reduction is facilitated by a well-rounded fitness regimen that includes both aerobic and strength training activities.

Consistency: Integrated into everyday life, consistent physical exercise is more beneficial for long-term fat reduction than intensive, irregular sessions.

Functional Movements: Working many muscle groups, including functional movements and exercises, improves overall fitness and encourages fat reduction.

4. Changes in behavior:

Goal Setting: Setting attainable, quantifiable, and time-bound objectives gives people direction and keeps them motivated.

Accountability: Having a personal trainer, a workout partner, or a supportive community might help you be more accountable and stick to your healthy routine.

Stress Management: Reducing stress with exercises like yoga, meditation, or deep breathing may help with fat reduction and stop stress-related overeating.

5. Enough Sleep:
Impact of Poor Sleep Quality: Hormonal imbalances caused by poor sleep have an impact on hormones that regulate hunger and raise the risk of weight gain.

Optimal Sleep Duration: To promote general health and aid in weight reduction, aim for 79 hours of good sleep per night.

Regular Sleep Schedule: By assisting in the regulation of circadian cycles, a regular sleep schedule may enhance the quality of one's sleep.

6. Surfactant:
Water Intake and Appetite: Maintaining a healthy fluid intake may help regulate appetite and avoid signals associated with dehydration that might be misinterpreted as hunger.

Replacing Sugary Beverages: Drinking water or other low-calorie beverages instead of sugary ones helps you consume fewer calories and lose weight.

7. Endocrine Balance:
Impact of Stress Hormones: Prolonged stress raises cortisol levels, which may lead to fat accumulation, particularly in the belly area.

Supporting Hormonal Health: Stress reduction, a healthy diet, and enough sleep all help to maintain hormonal balance, which supports long-term weight loss.

8. Personalized Methods:
Personalized Strategies: Developing successful fat reduction plans requires an understanding of how each person's metabolism, tastes, and lifestyle vary.

Consultation with Professionals: Consulting with dietitians, nutritionists, or fitness specialists can assist people in creating individualized plans that are in line with their particular requirements.

Genetic Considerations: Customized fat reduction techniques may be informed by knowledge of genetic characteristics that impact metabolism and sensitivity to various dietary regimens.

9. Sustained and Gradual Advancement

Avoiding Extreme Measures: Rapid weight reduction by drastic means often leads to rebound weight gain and muscle loss, highlighting the need for slow and steady progress.

Put Your Attention on Habits: Making the transition from short-term remedies to long-term habits will guarantee that weight reduction develops organically as a result of leading a healthy lifestyle.

Celebrate Non-Scale Victories: Maintaining motivation is facilitated by acknowledging accomplishments that go beyond the scale, such as more energy, a better mood, or higher fitness levels.

10. Empowerment in Education:

Nutritional Literacy: Improving nutritional literacy enables people to make knowledgeable food decisions, promoting a long-lasting and positive connection with food.

Understanding Metabolism: Busting misconceptions and fostering reasonable expectations for fat reduction are achieved by educating people about metabolism, including individual variances in it.

Difficulties and Things to Think About for Sustainable Fat Loss:

1. Myths and fallacies:
Spot Reduction Fallacy: denouncing the idea of spot reduction by highlighting the fact that focused fat loss in certain regions via exercise is not always successful.

Fast Fix Culture: Addressing the prevailing culture of fad diets and fast solutions, this initiative aims to raise awareness of the need for patience and dedication in order to achieve sustained weight reduction.

2. Analytical Elements
Body Image Concerns: Recognizing the influence of cultural norms on body image and fostering self-acceptance as an important element of the weight reduction process.

Diet Culture Influence: recognizing and questioning diet culture norms that might support unhealthful eating and body image interactions.

3. Hereditary Differenc
Individual Responses: Stressing the necessity for individualized methods, this statement acknowledges the variety in genetic responses to various food and exercise programs.

Metabolic Diversity: Being aware that hereditary variables might cause people to have different metabolic rates, which can affect how quickly they acquire or lose weight.

4. Environmental and social factors:

Social Pressures: Taking care of outside influences on body image and society norms that might affect people's drive to lose weight.

Environmental Influences: Being aware that social and physical environments might affect dietary and physical activity-related lifestyle decisions and behaviors.

5. Medical Conditions:

Medical Considerations: encouraging a holistic approach to health by recognizing and treating underlying medical disorders that may affect attempts to lose weight and fat.

Medication Influence: Understanding that certain drugs may alter metabolism or weight requires individualized approaches for each patient using a particular drug.

Next Developments in Long-Term Fat Loss:

1. Accurate Nutrition:

Personalized Dietary Recommendations: Developments in precision nutrition might result in very customized dietary advice depending on lifestyle, metabolic, and genetic variables.

Micro biome Interventions: Studies into how the gut micro biota regulates weight may open the door to microbial composition-focused therapies for enhanced fat reduction.

2. Integration of Digital Health:

Smart Technology Support: Ongoing incorporation of wearables and applications to track behaviors, provide real-time feedback, and encourage behavioral change.

Virtual Coaching Platforms: The emergence of artificial intelligence-powered virtual coaching platforms that provide tailored advice and assistance for long-term weight reduction.

3. Applications of Behavioral Psychology:
Behavioral Change Models: Improving adherence and motivation via the development and deployment of behavioral change models that address psychological aspects of weight reduction.

Gamified Wellness Programs: Adding gamification components to wellness initiatives to increase participant engagement and satisfaction with the weight loss process.

4. Healthy Weight Focus:
Metabolic Health Metrics: A move away from weight as the primary sign of successful fat reduction and toward metabolic health metrics such as inflammation and insulin sensitivity.

Comprehensive Health Assessment: For a more all-encompassing approach, fat reduction programs should include comprehensive health exams, which include hormone profiles and metabolic indicators.

5. Multidisciplinary Methods:
Cooperation among specialists: To provide complete fat reduction assistance, there is a growing level of cooperation among

nutritionists, fitness trainers, mental health specialists, and medical practitioners.

Integrated Health Platforms: The creation of integrated health platforms that unite specialists from different fields to handle the complex issues with fat reduction.

6. Initiatives Based on the Community:
Virtual Support Groups: Constant expansion of virtual groups devoted to long-term weight reduction, offering a forum for advice, inspiration, and experiences in common.

Community Wellness Programs: national and international campaigns that encourage participation in wellness activities within the community and build a sense of shared commitment to leading healthier lives.

7. Empowerment in Education:
Early Nutrition Education: To lay the groundwork for wholesome eating habits, educational initiatives encouraging nutritional literacy from a young age should be implemented.

Holistic Health Education: more extensive educational programs that highlight how emotional, mental, and physical health are all related to weight reduction.

Result:

Long-term weight reduction goes beyond traditional methods that just focus on restricting calories or engaging in intense physical activity. A comprehensive combination of precision nutrition, developments in digital health, applications of behavioral psychology, and multidisciplinary partnerships will be key to the future of fat reduction. Long-term success depends on recognizing the uniqueness of each journey, addressing cultural and psychological issues, and creating a supportive atmosphere.

As the field of fat reduction develops, the emphasis moves from seeking quick fixes to developing long-term lifestyle adjustments. The process becomes a combination of technical advancements, scientific discoveries, and people's empowerment to forge their own routes toward long-term weight reduction while exhibiting fortitude, self-awareness, and a comprehensive dedication to their general health and wellbeing.

Explaining Cross Fit Training

Unlocking Cross Fit's Power: Exercises, Concepts, and Transformative Fitness

CrossFit is a dynamic and very successful method of training that combines parts of weightlifting, gymnastics, aerobic exercise, and functional movements. This investigation explores the guiding concepts of CrossFit, the process used to create workouts, and the revolutionary effects it may have on people pursuing a variety of fitness objectives.

Cross-Fit Principles

The Fundamental Principles that Shape CrossFit's Approach to Fitness

CrossFit is a whole fitness philosophy based on ideas that go against conventional fitness conventions, not merely a set of exercises. Comprehending these fundamental principles offers discernment into the distinct methodology and perspective that characterize the CrossFit experience.

1. Regularly changing exercises:

Diverse activities: In order to minimize adaptation and promote overall fitness, CrossFit places a strong emphasis on exercises that are continuously varied and encompass a broad variety of functional activities.

Adaptation Challenge: Changing up your workouts on a regular basis forces your body to adjust to new stimuli, which keeps you from plateauing and maximizes your physical readiness.

2. Movements with Function:

Real-Life Applicability: CrossFit places a strong emphasis on functional exercises that mimic daily living activities, improving a person's capacity to carry out daily duties effectively and lowering their risk of injury.

Core to Extremity: A comprehensive and biomechanically sound approach to training is ensured by placing emphasis on using the core muscles before the extremities in motion.

3. Extremely intense exercises:

Efficiency and Intensity: CrossFit is distinguished by workouts that are high in intensity, with the aim of maximizing outcomes in a shorter amount of time via the performance of functional motions at a high intensity.

Adaptation Stimulus: High-intensity exercise promotes adaptation responses, which enhance cardiovascular health and result in increases in strength and endurance.

4. Observable and Measurable Outcomes:
Quantifiable Progress: CrossFit places a strong emphasis on outcomes that are quantifiable and visible, motivating participants to monitor their development over time.

Benchmark exercises: By including benchmark exercises, you can monitor progress consistently and objectively across a range of fitness disciplines.

5. Society and Friendship:
Group Dynamics: CrossFit promotes group exercise sessions that build a motivating and supportive atmosphere by fostering a sense of community.

Shared Goals: The friendships formed in CrossFit groups foster a shared dedication to reaching both personal and group fitness objectives.

6. Wide and all-encompassing fitness:
Adaptability: By preparing people for any physical challenge, whether in sports, emergency scenarios, or daily life, CrossFit fosters wide fitness.

Inclusivity: Because CrossFit exercises are scalable, people of all fitness levels, from novices to professional athletes, may participate.

7.   Eating right as the basis:
Holistic Approach: CrossFit acknowledges that diet plays a crucial role in maintaining general health and fitness.

Fueling Performance: It is believed that eating a healthy diet supports energy levels, promotes recuperation, and allows for peak performance throughout CrossFit exercises.

8.   Sport of CrossFit:
Competition Aspect: CrossFit has a competitive element, where top athletes may display their fitness prowess via events like the CrossFit Games.

Performance measures: Competitors in cross-fit events are judged on a range of performance measures, including strength, stamina, agility, and skill mastery.

Constructing CrossFit Exercises

The Science and Art of Creating Successful CrossFit Programs

Creating a cross-fit workout involves carefully balancing volume, intensity, and diversity of movements. It entails carefully planning the program to target several fitness domains and produce athletes who are versatile and well-rounded. CrossFit workouts are created using a science-based and artistic technique that takes into account the concepts of variety, scalability, and progression.

1. Thoughts on programming:

Goal Alignment: Determine the main fitness objectives to direct the entire program, such as increasing strength, cardiovascular endurance, agility, or a mix of these.

Progressive Overload: To encourage ongoing adaptation, use progressive overload by progressively increasing the volume, intensity, or complexity of your exercises.

2. Activity and WarmUp:

Dynamic WarmUp: To speed up heart rate, boost blood flow, and get the body ready for the exercise, start with a dynamic warmup.

Mobility Exercises: Include mobility exercises to improve joint range of motion and flexibility, which lowers the chance of injury while doing high-intensity workouts.

3. Components of strength:

Compound Movements: Include compound exercises like presses, deadlifts, and squats to work on large muscle groups and increase general strength.

Variety in Rep Schemes: Employ a range of repetition schemes, such as moderate repetition, moderate-weight exercises for muscular endurance, and low repetition, high-weight strength training.

4. Exercise for Metabolism (MetCon):

High-Intensity Intervals: MetCon increases heart rate and enhances cardiovascular fitness by including high-intensity intervals with little recovery time in between workouts.

Time and Rep Schemes: Both the anaerobic and aerobic energy systems are challenged by time-based exercises (such as AMRAP or as many rounds as possible) or prescribed repetitions with time limits.

5. Bodyweight and gymnastic movements:
Skill Development: To improve balance, body control, and spatial awareness, use gymnastics exercises like muscleups, pullups, and handstands.

Scalability: Offer scalable bodyweight exercise alternatives to suit people of all fitness levels, guaranteeing inclusion.

6. Weightlifting in the Olympics:
Technical Lifts: To improve power, speed, and coordination, use Olympic weightlifting exercises like snatches, cleans, and jerks.

Skill Emphasis: As participants become proficient in the technical components of weightlifting, the load will be progressively increased, with an emphasis on skill development.

7. Core Strengthening and Accessory Work:
Targeted Muscle Groups: Incorporate supplementary workouts to focus on certain muscle groups, correct imbalances, and enhance general athletic performance.

Core Stability: Include exercises that strengthen the core to provide stability, better posture, and more functional motions.

8. Recovery and Cooling Off:
Active Recovery: Include activities for active recovery to help reduce heart rate gradually and avoid blood pooling. This will speed up the healing process.

Stretching and Flexibility: To encourage muscular relaxation and increase range of motion, use static stretching and flexibility exercises.

9. Scheduling:
Cycles of Intensity: To maximize long-term performance and avoid burnout, use periodization by cycling between periods of high intensity and recuperation.

Skill Emphasis: Create exercises that, at different stages, concentrate on certain skills so that athletes may gradually become proficient with the motions.

10. Group and Community Exercises:
Team Challenges: Introduce team exercises that promote motivation and friendship among participants.

Community Events: To foster a feeling of camaraderie and mutual success, plan sporadic gettogethers or friendly contests.

11. Changes for Scaling:

Individual Adaptability: To provide an inclusive atmosphere, offer scaling alternatives for each exercise to suit people with different levels of fitness.

12. Programming with Particular Intentions:
Goal-Oriented Design: Customize programming to meet certain fitness objectives, such as competing better, gaining more strength, or increasing general fitness.

Periodic Assessments: Include periodic evaluations to monitor target progress and modify programming as necessary.

Difficulties and Things to Think About in CrossFit Training:

1. Prevention of injury:
Form Emphasis: To reduce the risk of injuries, particularly in high-intensity and complicated motions, emphasize appropriate form and technique throughout exercises.

tailored changes: To guarantee safe participation, coaches should be encouraged to provide tailored changes depending on participants' skills and limits.

2. Risks of Overtraining:
Rest and Recovery: Highlight the value of rest and recovery days in the CrossFit training regimen to reduce the danger of overtraining.

Pay Attention to Body Signals: To avoid overtraining, encourage participants to pay attention to their bodies and report any symptoms of exhaustion, pain, or discomfort.

3. Significant Difference

Fitness Levels: Recognize that there are a range of fitness levels in the CrossFit community and stress that exercises may be scaled to match the needs of all participants.

Skill Mastery: Acknowledge that everyone learns at a different pace, and some participants may need more time to master certain abilities.

4. Support for Nutrition:

Energy Demands: Draw attentions to the higher energy requirements associated with CrossFit exercise and inform participants of the value of a healthy diet in achieving their fitness objectives.

Hydration Emphasis: Stress the need to stay hydrated to maximize performance and promote recovery, particularly during intense exercises.

Upcoming Developments in CrossFit Training:

1. Integrated Technology:

Wearable Tech: Wearable technology is being integrated more and more to assess performance indicators, keep an eye on heart rate, and provide real-time feedback while working out.

Virtual Coaching Platforms: Technological developments in virtual coaching platforms that use artificial intelligence to assess movement patterns and provide tailored instruction.

2. Programming Driven by Data:
Performance Analytics: Enhancing performance analytics to monitor and assess each person's development would enable more accurate and data-driven programming.

Biometric input: Exercises may be customized depending on each person's unique physiological reactions by including biometric input, such as metabolic data and muscle oxygenation levels.

3. Integral CrossFit Courses:
Age-Specific Programs: Creation of customized CrossFit regimens that respond to the unique fitness requirements and concerns of various age groups.

Medical Condition Integration: Including CrossFit routines tailored for people with particular medical problems, with modifications, safety, and effectiveness in mind.

4. International Community Link:
Virtual Cross Fit Communities: The growth of online communities for Cross Fit that unite members worldwide and provide a sense of community despite distance.

International tournaments: more cooperation and involvement in international Cross Fit tournaments, fostering a more competitive and integrated worldwide community.

5. Including Mind Body Techniques:
The study aims to investigate the integration of mindfulness techniques into Cross Fit training as a means of improving mental resilience and attention during intense exercises.

Yoga and Mobility Fusion: To enhance flexibility, balance, and the mind-body connection overall, CrossFit incorporates yoga and mobility workouts.

6. Long-term Impact Research:
Longitudinal Studies: Researching the long-term effects of CrossFit training on a range of health parameters, including bone density, mental health, and cardiovascular health.

Injury Prevention Strategies: A constant study is being done to identify cross-fit injury prevention tactics that work, with the goal of improving procedures and standards to ensure safer participation.

7. Educational Materials:
Cross-Fit Certification Programs: Constantly evolving, these programs emphasize evidence-based techniques and have updated instructional materials.

available learning materials: creating online resources that are easily available to coaches and participants to inform them of the most recent developments in cross-fit training.

Result:

In the fitness business, CrossFit training is a paradigm shift that challenges traditional methods and promotes a dynamic, results-driven community. Its tenets—high-intensity exercises, functional motions, and a network of support—have transformed how people see and approach fitness objectives.

Exciting possibilities await CrossFit training in the future, from data-driven programming and technological breakthroughs to the continuous growth of a worldwide community bound by a common dedication to physical excellence. As CrossFit develops, the focus on injury prevention, inclusiveness, and holistic wellbeing will always be crucial, guaranteeing that people of all fitness levels may take advantage of this revolutionary approach to exercise. At the vanguard of a fitness revolution where innovation, camaraderie, and diversity come together for unmatched health and wellness results, CrossFit is inspiring both regular enthusiasts and top competitors.

Programs for Specialized Training

Unlocking the Potential: Power lifting Training Protocols and Endurance Events

Specialized training regimens focus on certain facets of physical performance while meeting targeted fitness objectives. In this investigation, we examine the nuances of training for endurance competitions as well as the power lifting training regimens that support the development of strength. Gaining an understanding of the guiding ideas, techniques, and factors involved in these programs may help people tailor their training to achieve specific fitness goals.

Endurance Event Training

Developing the Art of Endurance: Foundations and Techniques

Training for endurance events calls for a different kind of training that emphasizes mental toughness, stamina, and cardiovascular fitness. The concepts governing endurance training are essential for improving performance and getting the best outcomes, regardless of whether one is training for a long-distance bike ride, triathlon, or marathon.

1. Base Structure:

Aerobic Foundation: Building a strong aerobic base is the first step in endurance training. Activities that increase heart rate and improve oxygen use are emphasized.

Progressive Volume: Increase training volume gradually to develop endurance and help the body adapt to prolonged, sustained exertion.

2. Scheduling:

Training Cycles: Apply periodization by breaking the training program up into cycles that concentrate on various elements, including intensity, tapering, and base building.

Peaking Strategies: Make deliberate adjustments to training volume, intensity, and recovery in the runup to contests to optimize performance during particular events.

3. Training Specificity:

Sport Specific Activities: Adapt training to the demands of the particular endurance event by including, depending on the discipline, running, cycling, swimming, or a mix of these.

Terrain Considerations: Include training on surfaces that resemble the competition area if the event will take place on a variety of terrain.

4.   Runs with Intensity and Tempo:
Threshold Training: Increase your body's ability to withstand greater intensities for longer periods of time by including tempo and intensity runs.

Interval Training: To improve cardiovascular fitness and speed, use interval training, which alternates between periods of high-intensity exertion and active recuperation.

5.   Diet and Drinking Water:
Energy Requirements: Take care of the increased energy needs, emphasizing complex carbs as a long-lasting fuel source for workouts and competitions.

Hydration Strategies: Create hydration plans to avoid dehydration by taking the weather, the amount of exercise, and perspiration rates into account.

6.   Recuperation and Rest:
Importance of Rest: Acknowledge the role that rest days play in avoiding overtraining and in enabling the body to heal and adjust to the physiological strains that come with endurance training.

Active Recovery: To help muscles heal, include active recovery sessions that include low-intensity exercises like cycling or walking.

7. Emotional Sturdiness:

Mind-Body Connection: To overcome mental obstacles during extended physical endeavors, cultivate mental resilience via mindfulness exercises, visualization, and encouraging self-talk.

Race Simulation: Incorporate race simulations into your preparation to help you become more confident and comfortable while psychologically preparing for the difficulties of the real event.

8. Observation and Modifications:

Listen to the body: Assist athletes in recognizing fatigue indicators, tracking performance indicators, and modifying the training regimen in response to personal reactions.

Frequent evaluations: To monitor progress and modify training intensity appropriately, do frequent evaluations, such as time trials or fitness tests.

Difficulties and Things to Think About in Endurance Training:

1. Overuse Injury Risk:

Varied exercises: To lower the danger of overuse injuries brought on by repeated actions, including a range of endurance exercises,.

Correct Form Emphasis: To lessen the strain on joints and muscles during high-volume training, emphasize correct form and biomechanics.

2. Equilibrium Nutrition:

Individualized Nutrition: Recognize that every person has different nutritional demands and preferences; place an emphasis on a balanced diet that satisfies energy needs and aids in recuperation.

Avoiding Under fueling: Inform athletes about the risks of under fueling and stress the significance of consuming enough calories, particularly during times of rigorous exercise.

3. Emotional Tiredness:

Mental Recovery: In order to address mental exhaustion, include days of relaxation and mental-relieving activities that take your mind off the demands of endurance training.

Stress Management: Incorporate stress reduction methods, such as yoga or meditation, to lessen the mental strain brought on by extended training sessions.

4. Personal Rates of Adaptation:

Varied Responses: Be aware that various people react differently to endurance training and that, depending on your age, level of fitness, and experience, you may need to make adaptations.

Flexible Programming: Create training curricula that are adaptable to each person and may be changed in response to input and progress.

Upcoming Developments in Endurance Exercise:

Integrating Biometrics:
Wearable Tech Advances: The continuous incorporation of wearable technology to track biometric information, including oxygen saturation, heart rate variability, and hydration levels.

Real-Time Feedback: Personalized training session instruction is provided by real-time feedback systems that use biometric data.

Programs for Precision Training:
Genetic Considerations: Improvements in precision training regimens that take into account how a person's genetic makeup may affect how they react to certain endurance training stimuli.

Personalized Recovery Plans: Creating recovery plans that are specific to each person's reaction to training and take into account variables like stress levels and sleep quality.

Online Training Resources:
Virtual Training Environments: The development of immersive virtual training environments that replicate racing circumstances for athletes as a means of mental preparation.

Global Community Engagement: Establishing virtual communities that link endurance athletes worldwide, encouraging a spirit of friendship and common experiences.

Regarding the environment:
Climate-Specific Training: including training regimens tailored to a certain climate for athletes getting ready for endurance competitions in a range of environmental circumstances.

Altitude Training: Research into techniques for improving endurance performance at altitude, either in real-world or simulated situations.

Innovations in Recovery:
Cryotherapy Advancements: Technological developments in cryotherapy promote faster muscle repair, lessen inflammation, and improve recovery.

Nutritional Supplements: Studies on cutting-edge nutritional supplements created to meet the particular energy and recuperation requirements of endurance athletes.

Result: Strengthening Your Endurance

Training for endurance involves many different aspects and goes beyond just physical fitness; it also involves mental toughness, forethought, and flexibility. The combination of state-of-the-art technology, customized programming, and a worldwide community connection promises to redefine human performance limits as endurance training develops. Endurance sports need a harmonic fusion of science, creativity, and the unrelenting spirit of people who are dedicated to pushing the boundaries of what they can do.

Training Protocols for Power lifting

Power lifting Training: The Art and Science of Unleashing Strength

Pure strength is shown by power lifting, which calls for a unique training regimen that emphasizes the creation of maximum force. The concepts, exercises, and periodization techniques included in power lifting training regimens help competitors reach their maximum strength potential and succeed in the sport.

1. Principles of Foundations:
Maximal Strength Focus: Power lifting training emphasizes the capacity to lift the largest weights for a single repetition, with a focus on developing maximal strength.

Compound exercises: As the foundation of powerlifting training, give priority to compound exercises that hit the main muscular groups, such as the squat, bench press, and deadlift.

2. Strength Periodization:
Training stages: To maximize strength gains and performance, use periodization that advances through many stages, such as hypertrophy, strength, and peaking.

Manipulation of Volume and Intensity: Modify training volume and intensity at each phase, emphasizing hypertrophy to increase muscular mass, strength for maximum force, and peaking to prepare for competition.

3. Training Specificity:
Sport-Specific Movements: Design training to resemble the unique motions seen in power lifting contests, making sure that participants are ready for the squat, bench press, and deadlift.

Equipment Utilization: To improve performance and safety, use equipment designed specifically for powerlifting, such as lifting shoes, knee wraps, and belts.

4. Expertise in Technique:
Form Emphasis: To maximize force output and lower the risk of injury, emphasize good form and technique throughout powerlifting exercises.

Individualized Adjustments: Acknowledge that a person's anatomy may influence the best lifting technique; hence, minor modifications may be made in accordance with a particular athlete's biomechanics.

5. Strong Lifts and Gradual Overload:
maximum loads: To train the neuromuscular system for peak force output, use hard lifts with maximum loads while concentrating on low repetition ranges.

Progressive Overload: A key idea for ongoing strength development is to progressively increase the weight lifted over time in order to create progressive overload.

6. Complementary Activities:

Muscle Group Targeting: Include supplementary workouts that focus on certain muscle groups that assist powerlifting motions, resolving imbalances, and strengthening weak areas.

Variety in Movements: To target certain areas of strength development, use variants of the basic exercises, such as deficit deadlifts, closegrip bench presses, and stopped squats.

1. Recuperation and Rest:

Importance of Rest: Recognize the value of rest days in powerlifting training, as they enable the muscles and central nervous system to recuperate from strenuous lifting sessions.

Periodic Deloading: To avoid overtraining, lessen fatigue, and maximize performance in the following training cycles, implement periodic deloading weeks.

2. Diet for Sturdiness:

Caloric Surplus: To assist strength and muscle development, consider keeping a small surplus of calories, matching your diet to the energy requirements of powerlifting exercise.

Protein Intake: Make protein consumption a priority in order to aid in muscle repair and recuperation. Individual protein requirements should be met in accordance with exercise intensity.

3. Psychological Readiness:

Visualization Techniques: Use visualization techniques to practice successful lifts in your head, which will help you concentrate and feel more confident when competing.

Mindset Training: Cultivate a resilient mindset that welcomes obstacles, failures, and the strenuous mental strain of heavy lifting.

4. Simulation of competition:
Mock Competitions: Set up simulated training sessions or mock competitions that mimic the circumstances of a powerlifting meet to get athletes ready for the competitive setting.

Handling External Factors: Prepare athletes to deal with outside variables, including schedules, equipment rules, and the mentality of facing rivals.

Important Considerations and Obstacles in Powerlifting Training:

5. Dangers for Injury:
Load Management: To reduce the risk of overuse injuries brought on by regularly lifting large loads, emphasize appropriate load management.

Rehabilitation Protocols: To avoid exacerbations during training, implement rehabilitation protocols for any preexisting injuries and address them proactively.

6. Personal Reaction to Loudness:
Volume Sensitivity: Be aware that different people may react differently to training volumes; some people do better at lower volumes and higher intensities, while others do better at higher volumes.

Customized Programming: Create individualized training plans that take into account each athlete's rate of recuperation and adaptability to different training volumes.

7. Following Form Standards:
Judged Movements: Because powerlifting competitions include judged movements, make sure that competitors follow the particular form requirements for every lift.

Consistent Form Practice: To build muscle memory and reinforce correct technique for competition lifts, incorporate consistent form practice into your training sessions.

8. Psychological Stress:
Performance Anxiety: To help athletes manage stress during competitions, use techniques like mental preparation, positive self-talk, and visualization to address performance anxiety.

Handling Failures: Teach athletes how to accept failures in lifts and use them as teaching moments to advance their skills.

Upcoming Developments in Powerlifting Education:

9.   Analysis of Biomechanics:

Advanced Biomechanics: Make use of sophisticated biomechanical analysis methods to evaluate each person's lifting mechanics and offer suggestions for customized form modifications.

Biometric Feedback: To improve lifting mechanics and reduce injury risk, real-time biometric feedback is integrated into training sessions.

10. Technical Assistance:

Virtual Coaching Platforms: Technological developments in virtual coaching platforms that use artificial intelligence to assess lifting form, give tailored cues, and provide on-the-spot coaching.

The creation of wearable technology specifically for powerlifting, which records precise metrics like force production, bar speed, and lifting efficiency, is known as Wearable Tech Innovations.

11. Genetic points to remember:

Genetic Profiling: Investigation of potential genetic influences on an athlete's reaction to powerlifting training stimuli by means of genetic profiling.

Tailored Programming: Combining genetic data with programming to create individualized training plans according to a given athlete's genetic makeup.

12. Data-Driven Time Series Analysis:
The utilization of machine learning algorithms to evaluate training data and maximize strength gains through periodization strategies is known as "machine learning applications."

Individualized Peaking Protocols: To guarantee that athletes perform at their best during competitions, individualized peaking protocols are developed and adjusted based on data analysis.

13. Multidisciplinary Method:
Cooperation with Physiotherapists: enhanced cooperation with physiotherapists to apply all-encompassing strategies for injury prevention, such as mobility exercises and corrective exercises.

Nutrition and Recovery Support: Powerlifting training teams can benefit from the comprehensive support that nutritionists and recovery specialists offer for athletes' overall health.

14. Building the community:
Online Powerlifting Communities: Powerlifters around the world are feeling more connected as a result of the growth of online communities that promote knowledge sharing, peer support, and mentorship.

Social Media Impact: Social media platforms will continue to connect and amplify the voices of communities that lift weights, encouraging inclusivity and diversity in the sport.

as they surpass the capabilities of the human body.

Protocols for Powerlifting Training (Continued)

Cultural Influence:

Globalization of Powerlifting: Powerlifting is becoming more and more international, and this has led to a rise in participation from a wide range of cultural backgrounds. This has also influenced the development of training methods, which have been shaped by various lifting traditions.

Cultural Diversity in Training: This refers to acknowledging and incorporating various cultural viewpoints, which represent regional lifting styles, philosophies, and historical approaches, into powerlifting training.

Accessibility and Inclusivity:

Adaptive Powerlifting Programs: The creation of powerlifting programs that are tailored to the needs of people with disabilities in an effort to promote inclusivity and broaden the sport's appeal.

Accessible Equipment: Efforts to increase accessibility to powerlifting, such as the creation of facilities and equipment that can be adjusted to lift people of different sizes.

Whole-body Sports Development:
Mental Health Support: Powerlifting training programs now include mental health support services, recognizing the value of comprehensive athlete development.

Life Skills Education: programs that emphasize the importance of a comprehensive approach to athlete wellbeing by providing instruction in time management, stress management, and life skills.

Standards for Coaching and Education:
Enhanced Coaching Certification: Constant improvement of coaching certification programs with a focus on the most recent developments in strength and conditioning, evidence-based methods, and updated curriculum.

Accessible Education: Initiatives to improve the online accessibility of coaching education in order to give prospective coaches the tools they need to support the growth of powerlifting athletes.

Sustainability of the Environment:
Eco-Friendly Initiatives: The implementation of eco-friendly programs, such as waste reduction, energy-efficient practices, and sustainable equipment manufacturing, within powerlifting training facilities.

Green Certification: Powerlifting gyms that meet particular environmental sustainability standards are recognized and certified under this program, which encourages a conscientious approach to fitness.

Countermeasures:
Testing Advancements: To ensure the integrity of powerlifting competitions, there have been constant improvements made to antidoping measures. These include the use of more advanced testing techniques and closer cooperation with international antidoping agencies.

Clean Sport Education: Constant efforts to inform athletes, coaches, and support personnel about the significance of fair competition, the negative effects of doping, and clean sport principles.

Artificial Intelligence Integration:
AI-Powered Training Platforms: Powerlifting training platforms that incorporate artificial intelligence to provide customized workout suggestions, form analysis, and adaptive programming based on individual performance data.

Predictive Analytics: By using predictive analytics to identify possible areas for strength development, coaches and athletes can better tailor training regimens for the best possible outcomes.

The grassroots projects:
Youth Development Programs: community-based projects that introduced powerlifting to a younger audience and laid the groundwork for upcoming lifter generations.

Community Outreach: Powerlifting gyms that participate in outreach programs promote strength training, fitness, and healthy lifestyles outside of the competitive environment.

Collaboration in Scientific Research:
Universities and Research Centers: Powerlifting associations work with academic institutions to conduct research on biomechanics, nutrition, recuperation, and other aspects of strength training in order to continuously improve training techniques.

Data-Driven Insights: The sharing of information and understanding between researchers and the community of powerlifters, promoting a mutually beneficial partnership for evidence-based progress.

Initiatives for Social Impact:
Powerlifting for Social Causes: Including strength sports into larger societal initiatives by using powerlifting competitions and events to raise money and awareness for social causes.

Empowerment Programs: Establishing powerlifting initiatives to empower marginalized communities and advancing physical fitness as a means of fostering both individual and collective empowerment.

Result Changing Scene in Powerlifting:

As a sport and a way of life, powerlifting keeps changing to adapt to a changing environment. The powerlifting training landscape has been redefined through the integration of technological innovations, cultural diversity, and a holistic approach to athlete development. In addition to being a means of achieving physical prowess, sports also promote inclusivity, education, and constructive social impact.

Powerlifting is still based on the values of perseverance, discipline, and the neverending pursuit of individual and group strength objectives. Powerlifting is a dynamic force influencing the future of strength sports, regardless of whether athletes lift for competition, self-actualization, or community involvement. Powerlifting is a journey that involves more than just lifting weights; it also involves making an impact on people's lives, communities, and the state of fitness around the world.

Fitness Obstacles and Contests

Setting Out on the Expedition: Handling Fitness Difficulties and Contests

Fitness competitions and challenges provide people with a sense of community, structured goals, and the chance to push their physical and mental boundaries. These things act as catalysts for personal growth. Here, we explore the complexities of taking part in fitness challenges and training for competitions, revealing the many facets that characterize these life-changing experiences.

Starting Change: The Fitness Challenge Dynamics

Fitness challenges provide people with an exciting opportunity to jumpstart their wellness journey, overcome obstacles, and develop a regular physical activity habit. Fitness challenges, whether they are intended to promote weight loss, increased endurance, or general wellbeing, introduce an organized framework that encourages accountability, motivation, and a supportive community.

1. Choosing the Right Challenge:
Personal Alignment: Select a fitness challenge aligned with personal goals and interests, whether it's weight management, cardiovascular health, strength building, or a holistic approach encompassing multiple facets of fitness.

Realistic Timeframe: Consider the timeframe of the challenge, ensuring it aligns with individual commitments and allows for sustainable participation.

2. Goal Setting and Tracking:
SMART Goals: Establish Specific, Measurable, Achievable, Relevant, and Timebound (SMART) goals for the challenge, providing a clear roadmap for progress.

Tracking Mechanisms: Utilize tracking mechanisms such as fitness apps, journals, or wearable devices to monitor and measure progress throughout the challenge.

3. Community Engagement:

Online Platforms: Participate in online communities or forums related to the fitness challenge, fostering connections with likeminded individuals, sharing experiences, and gaining support.

Accountability Partners: Form accountability partnerships within the challenge community, creating a support system that encourages adherence to fitness goals.

4. Diversity in Activities:

Varied Workouts: Incorporate diverse workouts and activities to address different aspects of fitness, promote overall health, and prevent monotony.

Inclusion of Enjoyable Exercises: Include exercises and activities that bring joy, making the fitness journey more sustainable and enjoyable.

5. Nutritional Considerations:

Balanced Nutrition: Align nutritional choices with fitness goals, emphasizing a balanced diet that supports energy needs, muscle recovery, and overall wellbeing.

Education on Nutrition: Use the challenge as an opportunity to educate participants on nutrition principles, fostering a better understanding of the relationship between food and fitness.

6. Adaptability and Modifications:

Listen to the Body: Encourage participants to listen to their bodies and make necessary modifications to workouts or activities based on individual fitness levels and any physical limitations.

Program Flexibility: Design challenges with adaptable components, accommodating participants with varying fitness backgrounds, and allowing for inclusive participation.

7. Celebrating Milestones:
Recognition of Achievements: Celebrate individual and collective milestones achieved during the challenge, reinforcing positive behaviors and motivating continued effort.

Rewards and Incentives: Consider incorporating rewards or incentives for participants who achieve specific goals, enhancing motivation and commitment.

8. PostChallenge Reflection:
Evaluation of Progress: Facilitate a postchallenge reflection period, encouraging participants to evaluate their progress, identify lessons learned, and set new goals.

Transitioning to Long-Term Habits: Provide guidance on transitioning from the challenge into sustainable, long-term fitness habits, ensuring that the positive changes endure beyond the designated timeframe.

9. Overemphasis on Short-Term Goals:

Long-Term Perspective: Address the challenge of participants focusing solely on short-term goals by emphasizing the importance of adopting a long-term perspective for sustained health and fitness.

Education on Lifestyle Changes: Provide educational resources that underscore the significance of lifestyle changes beyond the challenge, encouraging participants to view fitness as an ongoing journey.

10. Potential for burnout:
Balanced Workouts: Mitigate the risk of burnout by promoting balanced workouts, allowing for rest days, and discouraging excessive exercise that may lead to fatigue.

Mental Well-Being: Incorporate components focusing on mental wellbeing within the challenge, including mindfulness activities or stress management techniques to support overall health.

11. Comparisons and self-esteem:
Individual Progress Emphasis: Shift the focus from external comparisons to individual progress, fostering a supportive environment that celebrates each participant's unique journey.

Body Positivity: Encourage body positivity and self-acceptance, promoting a healthy relationship with one's body and mitigating potential negative impacts on self-esteem.

12. Accessibility and Inclusivity:
Adaptable Challenges: Design challenges that are adaptable to various fitness levels, ensuring inclusivity and accessibility for individuals with different abilities and starting points.

Consideration for Diverse Participants: Address the diverse needs and preferences of participants, recognizing that a one-size-fits-all approach may not cater to everyone's individual circumstances.

Future Trends in Fitness Challenges:

13. Virtual Reality Integration:
Virtual Fitness Challenges: The integration of virtual reality (VR) technology with fitness challenges gives immersive experiences that imitate diverse activities, places, and training situations.

Worldwide Participation: virtual challenges that enable individuals from across the globe to participate in shared experiences, building a worldwide fitness community.

14. AIPowered Personalization:
AI-Driven Challenges: Development of challenges with AI-powered customization, customizing exercises, objectives, and feedback depending on individual preferences, performance, and progress.

Predictive Analytics: Use of predictive analytics to anticipate participants' requirements and personalize the challenge experience for optimum involvement.

15. Gamification Elements:
Gamified Challenges: Integration of gamification components, such as point systems, levels, and prizes, to boost participant motivation and pleasure.

Interactive Platforms: Development of interactive platforms that enable users to compete or cooperate digitally, providing a social and competitive aspect to fitness tasks.

16. Biometric Data Utilization:
Biometric Feedback Integration: Utilization of biometric data, obtained via wearable devices or sensors, to deliver real-time feedback, assess performance, and provide tailored insights.

Health Metrics Monitoring: The inclusion of health metrics monitoring inside challenges enables players to evaluate not just fitness progress but also wider health indicators.

17. Integration with Wearable Technology:
Wearable Tech Compatibility: seamless connection with wearable technology, allowing participants to sync their devices for precise tracking and real-time data exchange.

Health and Fitness Apps: Collaboration with prominent health and fitness apps to generate synergies between challenge platforms and existing monitoring programs.

Conclusion: The Evolution of Fitness Challenges

Fitness challenges have grown from basic physical assessments to full programs that target the complete wellbeing of participants. The future offers a combination of technological innovation, individualized experiences, and global connectedness, further strengthening the transformational influence of fitness challenges on people and communities.

Preparing for Fitness Competitions

Beyond Limits: The Art and Science of Competitive Fitness Preparation

Fitness contests represent the peak of physical performance, requiring precise preparation, dedication, and a comprehensive awareness of one's body. In the domain of competitive fitness, athletes experience a journey that stretches well beyond the gym, incorporating components of nutrition, mental fortitude, and strategic training to attain peak performance on competition day.

1. Understanding the Competitive Landscape:
    Investigating contests: Prioritize investigating and choosing contests that coincide with personal fitness objectives, including elements like format, judging criteria, and entry requirements.

Divisions and Categories: Familiarize yourself with the different divisions and categories within the competition, ensuring correct registration and preparation based on particular event conditions.

2. Periodized Training Approach:

Macro and Microcycles: Implement a periodized training technique, arranging training into macrocycles (long-term planning) and microcycles (short-term planning) to gradually peak on competition day.

Intensity and Volume Variation: Manipulate training intensity and volume across various stages, focusing strength, hypertrophy, and skill development according to competition needs.

3. Specialized Skills Development:

Sport-Specific Exercises: Incorporate sport-specific exercises and motions relevant to the competition, concentrating on honing abilities necessary for the particular events or challenges.

Technique Refinement: Dedicate training sessions to refining technique, ensuring ideal form and efficiency during competitive movements.

4. Nutrition Optimization:

Caloric and Macronutrient Planning: Develop a nutrition plan that matches training demands, providing adequate caloric intake and optimum macronutrient distribution to support energy requirements and recovery.

Meal Timing: Strategically arrange meals around training sessions and consider precompetition nutrition to improve performance and minimize energy depletion.

5. Recovery Strategies:
Active Recovery Methods: Implement active recovery methods, such as foam rolling, stretching, and low-intensity exercises, to enhance recovery between rigorous training sessions.

Sleep Prioritization: Prioritize appropriate sleep to assist in physical recovery, muscle restoration, and general wellbeing leading up to the competition.

6. Mental Preparation:
Visualization methods: Utilize visualization methods to mentally practice competing situations, boosting attention and confidence.

Stress Management: Develop stress management tactics to overcome precompetition anxieties and keep a collected mentality throughout the event.

7. Simulation and mock competitions:
Event Simulation: Incorporate simulated training sessions that closely mirror competitive situations, enabling athletes to practice pace, transitions, and mental resilience.

Mock contests: Organize mock contests to replicate the real event, offering a chance to identify possible obstacles and develop a strategy.

8. Acquaintance with Equipment:
Competition Specific Gear: Be sure you are comfortable and confident managing any equipment or gear that may be required for the competition.

Dresser Rehearsals: Utilize the competition equipment during training sessions to iron out any kinks and enhance performance.

9. Strategic Peaking
Tapering Protocols: To ensure the best possible recovery and performance, use tapering protocols in the last few weeks before the competition. These include progressively lowering training volume while maintaining intensity.

Peak Performance Timing: To prevent early peaking or performance decline, strategically schedule the peak of physical and mental preparedness to coincide with the competition date.

10. Technical and Usage Knowledge:
Reviewing Rules and Regulations: Become acquainted with the competition's rules and regulations to ensure that you follow them and avoid being disqualified.

Technical criteria: recognize any equipment specifications, form standards, and range of motion criteria that may apply to a particular event.

Difficulties and Things to Think About in Fitness Competitions:

Injury Risk Reduction:
Preventive Measures: Before increasing training intensity, give injury prevention a priority by doing mobility exercises, appropriate warm-ups, and treating any preexisting issues.

Adaptation Protocols: Create procedures that address recuperation and reduce the chance of aggravation when training is modified due to minor injuries.

Competitive Standards Adherence:
Constant Judging Criteria: During training, strive for constant adherence to competition standards while acknowledging the possibility of changes in judging criteria.

Incorporating Feedback: Adjust training to target areas for development and refine skills based on input from judges or seasoned competitors.

11. Emotional Sturdiness During the Contest:
Adapting to Unexpected Challenges: Provide athletes with mental resilience techniques so they can handle unforeseen

obstacles while competing while staying composed and focused.

Post-Event Reflection: Promote post-event reflection to assess performance, pinpoint takeaways, and cultivate a competitive mentality for future events.

Competitive Fitness Future Trends:

Digital Contests and Mixed Reality:
Virtual Event Platforms: The development of augmented reality-based virtual competition platforms that enable athletes to compete virtually while still preserving a competitive atmosphere.

AR Integration: Using augmented reality (AR) to provide a more futuristic and immersive visual representation of competition activities.

Performance Optimization Driven by Data:
Biometric Feedback Enhancement: Technological developments in biometric feedback systems that provide athletes access to real-time data during contests to help them maximize performance at the moment.

Performance Analytics: By using performance analytics to assess strengths and limitations, tailored training modifications are made possible for ongoing development.

International Cooperation and Titles:
United Global Events: The growth of global championships that unite athletes from many nations in large-scale fitness competitions.

International Collaborations: A greater degree of cooperation among international fitness groups has led to the standardization of competition rules and formats.

Including Esports Components:
Esports Components in Fitness: Including esports components in fitness contests to combine real-world gaming with virtual skills.

Interactive Spectator Engagement: Creation of interactive systems that enable online interaction, real-time discussion, and even hands-on involvement in certain competition areas.

Final Thoughts: The Prospects for Competitive Fitness:

At the nexus of athleticism, strategy, and innovation lies competitive fitness. The future of competitive fitness will be redefined as the environment changes due to the integration of cutting-edge technology, worldwide cooperation, and creative training approaches. Athletes may expect a constantly changing competitive field, shaped in part by data-driven insights, AI-supported coaching, and virtual tournaments.

Concluding Remarks Regarding Fitness Competitions and Challenges:

Participating in fitness challenges and contests is a life-changing experience that involves mental toughness, tactical preparation, and a dedication to ongoing progress. It's not only about hitting physical goals. People go on quests that take them outside of the gym, whether they are preparing for a competitive event or taking part in a community fitness challenge.

These contests and challenges serve as venues for introspection and encourage participants to reach new limits with their talents. Future predictions and changing trends suggest that technology will keep finding its way into the fitness industry, creating a worldwide network of athletes who are all passionate about being physically exceptional.

One thing never changes as we traverse this evershifting landscape: the spirit of competitiveness entwined with the quest for personal development. Every participant, whether setting a new personal record in a fitness challenge or competing, adds to the collective story of a worldwide fitness community that values commitment, creativity, and the unwavering pursuit of peak performance.

Building a Home Workout Center: Strengthening Your Fitness Path

Constructing a Strength and Wellness Sanctuary

The idea of a home gym has been quite popular recently since it gives people the freedom to work out whenever it's convenient for them and in a setting that suits their tastes. Building a home gym is more than just putting equipment together; it's about designing a haven that inspires, encourages, and integrates into daily life. In this investigation, we explore the fundamentals of setting up a home gym, from choosing the appropriate equipment to creating a functional training area.

Crucial Home Exercise Equipment

Building Your Fitness Armoury: Essential Home Gym Equipment

The first step in creating a functional home gym is to carefully choose equipment that optimizes available space, supports a variety of training styles, and is in line with personal fitness objectives. This is a thorough reference to the fundamental tools that make up a well-rounded home gym:

Equipment for Cardiovascular Exercise:
Treadmill: Suitable for aerobic exercises, a treadmill provides the ease of walking or jogging in the comfort of your own home while enhancing cardiovascular endurance.

Stationary Bike: A stationary bike burns calories and improves cardiovascular fitness while providing low-impact cardio, which makes it appropriate for those with joint difficulties.

Elliptical Trainer: A flexible option for home gyms, an elliptical trainer combines aspects of running and cycling to provide a full-body exercise with low pressure on joints.

Equipment for strength training:
Dumbbells: Suitable for a wide range of strength training exercises, dumbbells enable users to target certain muscle areas and gradually build resistance. They are also space-efficient and versatile.

Kettlebells: By combining dynamic motions that work many muscle groups and improve functional strength and flexibility, kettlebells bring variation to strength training.

Resistance Bands: A less expensive option to standard weights, resistance bands are small, versatile, and give different degrees of resistance for workouts involving the upper and lower bodies.

Adjustable Weight Bench: By enabling a variety of exercises, such as rows, chest presses, and seated workouts, an adjustable weight bench enhances strength training.

Equipment for bodyweight and functional training:

Medicine Ball: Adding a dynamic aspect to at-home workouts, medicine balls improve core strength, stability, and coordination via their use in dynamic exercises.

Suspension Trainer (e.g., TRX): By using body weight as resistance, a suspension trainer allows for a variety of bodyweight workouts that improve balance, strength, and flexibility.

Pull-Up Bar: By installing a pull-up bar in a doorway, one may work out their upper body in an efficient manner, working their arms, back, and core with exercises like leg raises and chinups.

1. Tools for Flexibility and Recovery:
Yoga Mat: A comfortable, nonslip yoga mat improves comfort and hygienic conditions during exercise by providing a base for floor exercises, yoga, and stretching regimens.

Foam Roller: By reducing muscular tension and increasing flexibility, a foam roller helps with self-myofascial release and facilitates muscle healing.

Yoga Blocks and Straps: Yoga blocks and straps help with good alignment and deeper stretches for those who include them in their regimen.

2. Technology and surveillance equipment:
Smart Fitness Tracker: By tracking vital signs like heart rate, steps, and calories burned, wearable fitness trackers provide insightful data on daily activity and advancement.

Smartphone or Tablet: To mix up your exercises and maintain motivation, use fitness applications, online workout plans, and educational videos on your Smartphone or tablet.

TV or Mirror: Installing a TV or mirror in the home gym area makes it easier to follow along with exercise videos and guarantees correct form and technique.

3. Organization and Storage Solutions:
Equipment Rack or Shelving: Reduce clutter in your home gym by adding racks or shelves to hold weights, resistance bands, and smaller accessories.

MultiFunctional Storage Bench: A storage bench serves as a space-saving, dual-purpose solution by serving as both a seat for workouts and equipment storage.

4. Comfort and Hydration Needs:
Water Dispenser or Bottle: Having a water dispenser or a specialized water bottle makes it easier to get refreshment during exercises, which emphasizes the need to stay hydrated.

Cooling Fan or Ventilation: Make your home gym more comfortable by adding a cooling fan or making sure there is enough ventilation.

5. Attractions and Inspirational Aspects:
Bluetooth Speakers: Play upbeat music on Bluetooth speakers to set the mood for your exercises and improve your overall performance.

Inspiration Wall: Arrange inspirational sayings, exercise objectives, or pictures that encourage and strengthen dedication to the fitness path on an inspiration wall.

Choosing Gear According to Fitness Objectives:

Regarding cardiovascular health:
Top Gear: elliptical trainer, stationary cycle, and treadmill.

Additional Options: For variation, try an aerobic stepper, a rowing machine, or a jump rope.

For developing strength and muscle:
Dumbbells, kettlebells, and an adjustable weight bench are the priority pieces of equipment.

Extra Options: power rack, squat stand, or barbell and plates.

Training in Flexibility and Functionality:
Yoga mats, resistance bands, and suspension trainers are the top priorities.

Stability balls, foam rollers, and medicine balls are additional options.

For General Well-Being and Recuperation:
The foam roller, yoga mat, and water station are the priority equipment.

Additional options: massage equipment, aromatherapy diffusers, and comfy chairs.

Creating an Efficient Home Gym Area Converting a Room into a Fitness Sanctuary: Creating the Ideal Home Gym Ambience

Planning carefully is necessary to maximize utility, atmosphere, and motivation when creating a home gym. Whether you have a dedicated space or a little nook, thoughtful planning may improve your entire home-based workout experience.

Selecting the appropriate site:
Assess Available Places: Examine the places in your house that are available, taking into account garages, basements, extra rooms, or even repurposing a corner of a living room or bedroom.

Natural Light and Ventilation: To create a warm and stimulating environment, choose a room with enough natural light and ventilation, wherever feasible.

Attention to Flooring:
Shock-absorbing Flooring: Make an impact-absorbing flooring purchase, particularly if you use jumps or heavy lifting as part of your exercises. Specialized gym mats, interlocking tiles, and rubber floors are available options.
Easy to Clean: Choose flooring that is simple to keep clean and maintain to guarantee a sanitary working environment.

Arrangement and Structure:
Functional Zones: Assign certain zones for strength, flexibility, and cardio routines. Set up your equipment so that there is flow and less congestion.

Storage Solutions: To keep equipment accessible and organized, use storage solutions like bins, shelves, and racks.

Showers and Eye Appeal:
Full-length Mirrors: Install full-length mirrors to create a visually open and reflecting atmosphere while monitoring form and posture during workouts.

Aesthetic Elements: To personalize the area and increase motivation, add aesthetic elements like plants, motivational posters, or ornamental accents.

Control of Temperature and Ventilation:
Assure Adequate Ventilation: Install fans or make sure there is enough ventilation to keep the gym pleasant, particularly during long workouts.

Temperature Regulation: To guarantee a comfortable exercise, take into account the room's temperature and use heating or cooling solutions.

Design of Lighting:
Natural and Artificial Lighting: To guarantee well-lit training sessions that enhance attention and safety, balance natural light with thoughtful placement of artificial lighting.

Changeable lighting: To accommodate varying exercise intensities and provide a dynamic atmosphere, if at all feasible, use changeable lighting.

Hardware Configuration:
High-Quality Speakers: To enjoy music, educational films, or virtual courses, invest in high-quality speakers or sound systems, which will improve the environment overall.

Soundproofing Considerations: To reduce noise annoyance to other occupants of the house, take into account soundproofing techniques if your home gym is in a common area.

Security and Noise-Free Area:
Minimize Distractions: To establish a focused and committed exercise atmosphere, move the home gym away from busy areas and reduce distractions.

Privacy Screens or Curtains: To establish a dedicated training area in a common gym, think about using privacy screens or curtains.

Safety and accessibility:
Emergency Exit Access: Make sure that, in the event of a safety risk, there is simple access to emergency exits and clear paths.

Safety Flooring: Put safety first by selecting flooring that reduces the possibility of trips and falls, particularly in locations where perspiration buildup is common.

Technological Integration:
Secure Tech Mounting: Make sure that any technology—such as a TV, tablet, or Smartphone—is mounted securely to avoid mishaps while working out.

Accessible Outlets: Organize outlets such that they can power electronics without putting people in danger from tripping over extension wires.

Adaptability for Various Uses:
Convertible Furniture: Take into account pieces of furniture that are readily movable or modified to suit different tastes and methods of exercise.

Foldable Equipment: If available space is restricted, use foldable or collapsible equipment to maximize flexibility in using your home gym.

Consistent upkeep and cleaning:
Scheduled Cleaning Routine: Create a schedule for keeping your home gym clean and sanitary so that it's a welcoming and hygienic place to work out.

Equipment Inspection: To guarantee lifespan and safety, regularly examine and repair exercise equipment.

Inspiration and Personalization:
Motivational Wall: To maintain motivation, designate a wall area for recording progress, writing motivational sayings, and setting fitness objectives.

Personal Touch: To make the room really yours, add personal elements like artwork, colors, or décor that speak to your fitness journey.

Online Communication:
Strong WI-Fi Signal: If you want to participate in virtual training, courses, or streaming services, make sure you have a strong and steady Wi-Fi signal for uninterrupted access.

Charging Stations: To keep electrical gadgets charged while working out, set up charging stations.

Growth and Flexibility:
Modular Design: Choose a layout that will enable the home gym to be expanded or modified in the future as your exercise demands change.

Adaptable Storage: Select storage options that are simple to reorganize to make room for new equipment or evolving fitness tastes.

Important Factors and Difficulties in Designing Home Gyms:

Restricted Area:
Space-efficient Equipment: Prioritize multipurpose and compact equipment to make the most use of the available space.

Vertical Storage Solutions: To maximize floor space, use vertical space for equipment installation and storage.

Communal Living Areas:
Schedule and Communication: To reduce disputes during exercise times, establish clear timetables and lines of communication with other members of the family.

Portable Equipment Options: For shared locations, think about storing or bringing portable equipment that can be quickly put up and taken down.

Fiscal Restrictions:
Prioritize Essentials: Set aside money for necessary gear initially, then progressively increase it in accordance with your fitness objectives and financial resources.

DIY Solutions: To save expenses, consider DIY or repurposed options for components like storage, organization, or décor.

Natural light is limited.
Strategic Lighting Solutions: To make up for inadequate natural light, strategically use artificial lighting solutions, such as brilliant LED lights.

Mirrors for Reflection: Make use of mirrors in a strategic manner to reflect ambient light and make an area seem brighter.

Future Directions for Designing Home Gyms:

Smart Home Workout Compatibility:
AI-Powered Workouts: Utilizing artificial intelligence to provide form correction, progress monitoring, and customized exercise suggestions.

Smart Gym Equipment: Development of gym equipment with built-in connections, enabling data synchronization with fitness applications and virtual coaching platforms.

Fitness for Virtual Reality:
VR-Enhanced Workouts: Utilizing virtual reality (VR) technology to create immersive workouts that mimic different settings and situations.

Interactive VR fitness courses: real-time involvement in virtual fitness courses that foster a sense of community and teacher direction.

Design of Sustainable Gyms:
Eco-Friendly Equipment: Promoting environmentally responsible exercise habits by expanding the availability of sustainable and eco-friendly home gym equipment.

Green Building Materials: Utilizing sustainable and energy-efficient building materials while constructing home gyms.

Integrating Biometrics:
Biometric Feedback Systems: Improved biometric feedback system integration into home gym designs, including performance data and real-time health indicators for customized training modifications.

Biometric Recognition Equipment: The creation of fitness equipment with integrated biometric recognition technology enables smooth monitoring and personalization according to user data.

Hybrid Exercise Programs and Multipurpose Areas:
Adaptable Furniture: Ongoing innovation in multipurpose, adaptable furniture that switches between training and nonworkout modes with ease.

Interactive Workout Surfaces: Adding interactive surfaces that may alter resistance or texture increases the adaptability of exercise areas.

Help with Augmented Reality Fitness:
AR Workout Coaching: Augmented reality is being used to provide interactive visualizations, overlays of exercise instructions, and real-time workout coaching.

AR-Enhanced Equipment: Augmented reality elements provide a dynamic and engaging element to gym equipment.

Personalized digital environments:
Personalized Workout Environments: Users may personalize virtual landscapes and energetic cityscapes to fit their workout tastes.

Gamified Fitness Challenges: virtual settings with gamification components to increase the engagement and motivation of exercise.

Online Fitness Mentoring:
Remote Personal Trainers: An increasing number of remote personal trainers are available to provide people with individualized instruction from any location on the globe.

AI-Powered Virtual Coaches: The incorporation of artificial intelligence-powered virtual coaches who evaluate performance, adjust form, and modify exercises in response to real-time data.

Final Thoughts: The Future Home Gym:

The development of home gym design offers an exciting blend of technology, sustainability, and tailored wellbeing as we navigate an era when home fitness takes center stage. The modern home gym is more than just a physical area; it's a dynamic ecosystem that incorporates state-of-the-art technologies, conforms to personal tastes, and encourages a whole-person approach to wellness.

The home gym of the future will be a place where exercises are guided by AI-powered coaches, training becomes an immersive experience thanks to virtual reality, and eco-friendly practices complement eco-conscious lives. It will fit right in with our everyday routines and provide a safe sanctuary for our physical and emotional health.

Whether you are designing a home gym now or in the future, the secret is to be flexible, plan ahead, and be dedicated to creating a place that supports your fitness quest. The home gym is an investment in a way of life that places a premium on flexibility, health, and being the best version of oneself rather than merely a reflection of the latest fashions.

Maintaining Physical Fitness throughout Life: Promoting Overall Wellness

Discovering the Fountain of Youth with Personalized Exercise

The dynamic interaction between aging and fitness has a substantial impact on people's wellbeing as they go through various phases of life. Keeping up and making adjustments to one's fitness regimen becomes essential for living a happy and healthy life, regardless of age. In this investigation, we explore the subtleties of age-appropriate fitness, illuminating the advantages of exercise, particularly for the elderly.

Achieving the Specific Requirements of Each Stage

1. Adolescence and Youth: Establishing Bases for a Lifetime of Health

Focus on Fundamentals: For young people, the development of basic movement patterns, enhancement of coordination, and establishment of a solid basis for future fitness endeavors should be prioritized.

Diverse Physical Activities: Promote involvement in a range of physical activities, such as sports, dancing, and leisure games, to cultivate a love of movement and social interaction.

Strength and Flexibility Training: To improve joint mobility, muscular growth, and general physical resilience, introduce fundamental strength and flexibility training.

2. "Adulthood: Juggling Personal Fitness, Family, and Career"

Incorporate Regular Cardiovascular Exercise: To promote heart health and sustain energy levels, individuals with hectic schedules should concentrate on incorporating regular cardiovascular workouts like cycling, swimming, or running.

Strength Training for Longevity: Maintain muscle mass, support bone health, and fend off the aging process's natural loss of muscle mass by doing strength training.

Stress-Relieving Hobbies: To balance the pressures of work and family obligations, including stress-relieving hobbies like yoga or mindfulness exercises,.

3. Middle Ages: Handling Transitions and Giving Health First Priority

Flexibility and Mobility Work: Regular flexibility and mobility exercises may help avoid injuries and promote joint health by combating stiffness and restricted range of motion.

Combination of Cardio and Strength: To maintain a healthy weight, control stress, and lower the risk of chronic illnesses linked to aging, combine cardiovascular activities with strength training.

Regular Health Screenings: Make routine health examinations and screenings a priority in order to identify and treat any health problems early on and promote proactive wellbeing.

4. Older People: Maintaining Vitality and Self-Sufficiency

Low-Impact Cardiovascular Activities: To promote heart health without overstressing joints, use low-impact cardiovascular exercises like swimming, strolling, or stationary cycling.

Functional Strength Training: Put an emphasis on functional strength training, which focuses on improving independence, addressing activities of daily living, and lowering the risk of falls.

Exercises for Balance and Flexibility: Incorporate these types of activities into your routine. They are essential for preserving mobility and avoiding injuries that are frequent among seniors.

Senior Exercise Benefits

Unlocking the Fountain of Youth: Maintaining Good Physical and Mental Health in Later Life

1. Better cardiovascular conditions:

Improved Blood Circulation: Reducing the risk of cardiovascular illnesses and boosting heart health, regular exercise encourages healthy blood circulation.

Blood Pressure Management: Exercise helps control blood pressure, which helps ward off hypertension and its aftereffects.

Enhanced Cardiovascular Endurance: Seniors who exercise their cardiovascular systems have better endurance, which gives them more stamina for everyday tasks.

2. Preserving Bone Density and Muscular Strength:
Preservation of Muscle Mass: By preventing the aging-related natural loss of muscle mass, strength training activities enhance functional strength.

Bone Health: Resistance and weightbearing workouts promote bone density, which lowers the incidence of osteoporosis and fractures in the elderly.

Joint Health: Mild joint strengthening activities relieve stiffness and soreness while preserving joint flexibility.

3. Enhanced Stability and Prevention of Falls:
Improved Balance: Seniors who engage in balance exercises, such as heel-to-toe walking or standing on one leg, report feeling more stable and experiencing fewer falls.

Fall Prevention Strategies: Strength training and balancing exercises improve proprioception and coordination, two vital components of fall prevention.

Increased Confidence: Seniors who regularly exercise to maintain excellent balance often report feeling more confident in their day-to-day activities.

4. Academic Advantages:
Brain Health: Studies on the relationship between exercise and age-related cognitive decline have shown improvements in cognitive performance.

Memory Enhancement: Seniors who regularly exercise may have improved cognitive and memory functions.

Mood Regulation: Exercise lowers the risk of depression and anxiety in older individuals by releasing endorphins, which help to regulate mood.

5. Metabolic Health and Weight Management:
Healthy Weight Maintenance: By boosting a healthy metabolism and burning calories, regular exercise helps people maintain a healthy weight.

Blood Sugar Regulation: Exercise promotes general metabolic health and lowers the risk of diabetes by helping to manage blood sugar levels.

Insulin Sensitivity: Regular exercise raises insulin sensitivity, which is crucial for senior diabetes prevention and management.

6. Management of Arthritis and Joints:
discomfort relief: Seniors with arthritis-related joint discomfort may find relief from low-impact activities like swimming or cycling.

Joint Mobility: Preserving joint mobility with mild exercise reduces stiffness and pain while improving general joint health.

Adapted Exercise Programs: Seniors may participate in physical activity in a safe and comfortable manner with specially designed exercise programs that take into account their unique joint issues.

7. Emotional Health and Social Participation:
Community Involvement: Taking part in fitness courses or group exercise sessions encourages social interactions, which lessens the sense of loneliness that many seniors experience.

Emotional Resilience: Regular exercise helps foster emotional resilience and a positive mindset, which are important coping skills for overcoming obstacles in life.

feeling of success: Maintaining an active lifestyle and reaching fitness goals provide a feeling of purpose and success that enhances mental health in general.

8. Improved Quality of Sleep:
Sleep Regulation: By controlling circadian cycles and easing the symptoms of insomnia, exercise helps people sleep better.

Deeper Sleep: Seniors who regularly exercise often have deeper, more restful sleep, which improves their general wellbeing.

Sleep length: Research has shown that physical exercise enhances sleep length, which supports older people's healthy sleep habits.

Including Seniors in Safe Exercise:

9. Healthcare Professional Consultation:
PreExercise Health Check: Seniors, particularly those with preexisting medical issues, should see their healthcare practitioner for a preexercise health check.

Medication Considerations: Talk to medical specialists about possible interactions between drugs and exercise.

10. Adaptations and Gradual Progression:
Start Slowly: To prevent overexertion, start with low-intensity exercises and work your way up to more difficult ones.

Adaptations for Physical Limits: To guarantee safety and pleasure, modify workouts depending on physical limits or medical issues.

11. WarmUp and Cool Down: WarmUp Routine: Warm up your muscles and joints before working out to get them ready for action. This might include joint mobility exercises, mild aerobic workouts, and stretches.

Cool-down Practices: Following your exercise, stretch your body to increase flexibility and help it gradually become relaxed.

12. Diet and Hydration:
Hydration Awareness: To promote general health and avoid dehydration, seniors should be encouraged to drink enough water before, during, and after physical activity.

Balanced Nutrition: Stress the value of eating a nutritious, well-balanced diet that includes enough protein for healthy muscles and calcium for strong bones.

13. Continuous Observation and Modifications:
Self-monitoring: Assist elders in observing how their bodies react to physical activity and noting any pain or odd symptoms.

Modification of Intensity: Be willing to modify the kind and degree of exercise in accordance with personal comfort levels and any changes in health condition.

14. Group Activities and Social Support:
Enrolling in group fitness programs: Group fitness programs provide a feeling of camaraderie, motivation, and social support.

Family and Friends Involvement: To foster a positive and joyful atmosphere, encourage family members or friends to participate in joint physical activities.

Next Developments in Senior Exercise:

15. Online Fitness Resources:
Online fitness sessions: More senior-focused online fitness sessions are becoming available, offering accessibility and flexibility.

Virtual Reality Training Programs: By incorporating virtual reality into training routines, exercises become more entertaining and participatory.

16. Adaptive Technologies:
Smart Devices for Monitoring: Ongoing development of smart devices with capabilities for emergency response, health monitoring, and advice tailored especially for elders.

Wearable Technology for Seniors: wearable gadgets with graphical user interfaces that are tailored to the particular requirements of elderly people and encourage active aging.

17. Fitness Programs for All Generations:

Community-Based Initiatives: supporting fitness programs that bridge generations by bringing older and younger people together for shared exercise.

Fitness Challenges for All Ages: Senior participation in fitness competitions and activities promotes a feeling of accomplishment and community engagement.

18. Personalized Fitness Plans for Long-Term Illnesses:
Specialized Programs: Creation of fitness regimens tailored to elderly patients with long-term health issues, including diabetes, cardiovascular disease, or arthritis.

Integration of Rehabilitation Methods: Seniors with mobility issues or post surgery recovery requirements might benefit from the integration of rehabilitation methods into exercise programs.

19. Fitness Technologies for Home Use:
Interactive Home Exercise Systems: An increasing number of personalized, real-time feedback interactive home exercise systems are available.

AI-Powered Virtual Trainers: Using artificial intelligence, customized virtual trainers that can modify exercises according to each user's progress and health state have been created.

Result: Aging in a Graceful Way with Movement:

Fitness and aging go hand in hand, demonstrating the transforming potential of exercise in fostering both physical and emotional wellbeing. People have a canvas on which to paint their fitness story, changing and growing with each stage of life, from youthful enthusiasm to the wisdom of old age.

With customized exercise, seniors, in particular, have the key to opening the fountain of youth. Staying physically active has many advantages, but it also improves social interaction, emotional stability, and cognitive function.

Looking forward, the senior exercise scene offers a well-balanced mix of technology, diversity, and individualized wellbeing. Seniors are positioned to rewrite the story of aging gracefully via movement, whether they choose to use adaptive technology, engage in intergenerational fitness programs, or embrace virtual reality exercises.

The pursuit of health and aging is a celebration of the resiliency and growing potential of the human soul. It is evidence that pursuing wellbeing is a lifelong activity that never goes out of style and that every breath, walk, and stretch adds to a life well lived.

Sport-Specific Training: Using Precision and Variety to Improve Athletic Performance

Creating Excellence with Each Motion

The ultimate level of athletic preparation is achieved through sport-specific training, where people are shaped into finely tuned athletes through a combination of accuracy and variety. This investigation explores the complexities of improving athletic performance with customized and varied fitness routines, including everything from the minute details of training for a specific activity to the tactical benefits of cross-training.

19.1 Sports-Specific Training

Discovering the Keys to Excellence in a Particular Sport

1. Knowing the particular requirements
   Deconstructing Sport Motions: Creating a tailored training program begins with examining the basic motions and demands of a particular sport.

   Identifying Muscle Groups: Athletes may focus their training efforts on improving the strength, endurance, and flexibility necessary for peak performance by identifying the muscle groups used in certain sport-specific motions.

   Skill-Based Training: Including skill-specific exercises in the training program helps to improve coordination, perfect technique, and develop muscle memory—all of which are essential for success in the chosen sport.

2. Scheduling to Achieve Peak Performance:
Macro and Microcycles: Applying periodization entails dividing training into long-term (macrocycle) and short-term (microcycle) training plans, maximizing training loads, and adding recovery intervals to reach competitive peak times.

Pre-, in-, and off-season training focused on the stage of the season guarantees athletes' physical and mental readiness for the unique demands of competition.

3. Building Strength and Power:
Explosive motions: Training that emphasizes motions that resemble the swift and forceful moves needed during competition is beneficial for sports like weightlifting, basketball, and sprinting.

Sports Specific Resistance Training: Including resistance exercises that mimic motions unique to a certain activity improves functional strength, which in turn leads to better performance.

Adaptations for Endurance Activities: Strength training helps maintain posture, avoid injuries, and increase muscular endurance in activities that emphasize endurance.

4. Conditioning of the Heart:

Aerobic and Anaerobic Training: In order to fulfill the unique demands of competition, cardiovascular training should balance the aerobic and anaerobic components to address the energy systems that are prominent in the sport.

Interval Training: By simulating the intensity swings of several sports, intervals improve cardiovascular fitness and allow athletes to exert significant effort over extended periods of time.

Altitude Training: To improve oxygen usage and endurance in sports where altitude is a factor, simulated altitude training may be used.

5. Dexterity and adaptability

Agility Drills: Activities that enhance rapid direction changes, balance, and response times are beneficial for sports like basketball, tennis, and soccer.

Dynamic Flexibility Training: Combining sport-specific dynamic stretches and motions improves flexibility and gets muscles ready for the dynamic activities that competitors face.

Activity-specific yoga or Pilates, including exercises that are tailored to a particular activity, improves flexibility, core strength, and body awareness, all of which improve overall athletic performance.

6. Integrating Sport Psychology:

Visualization Techniques: Mental training is just as important as physical training. Through the mental practice of sport-specific situations, visualization methods help players improve their attention and confidence.

Stress Management: Psychological resilience training helps athletes learn how to control their stress, remain composed under duress, and cultivate an optimistic outlook.

Goal Setting: Athletes have a clear path to success when they set SMART (specific, measurable, attainable, relevant, and time-bound) objectives.

7. Recuperation Techniques:
PostTraining Nutrition: Refueling energy reserves and accelerating muscle regeneration are achieved by customizing nutrition to promote recovery, including the correct ratio of macro and micronutrients.

Optimization of Sleep: Setting aside time for restorative sleep is crucial for promoting the physical and mental renewal needed for long-term performance.

Active Recovery Techniques: Including low-intensity exercises on recovery days, such as swimming or cycling, improves blood flow, eases stiffness in the muscles, and promotes general healing.

8. Testing and Monitoring Particular to Sports:
Performance measurements: Coaches and players may assess progress and pinpoint areas for growth by using

sports-specific performance measurements, such as sprint timings, agility exercises, or endurance benchmarks.

Technology Integration: Using GPS trackers, wearables, or biomechanical analysis tools provides real-time data that may be used to precisely modify training methods.

Regular fitness exams, which include flexibility testing, cardiovascular evaluations, and strength tests, help shape training regimens as they are developed.

9. Scheduling of Nutrients

Energy Demands: By understanding how various sports need different amounts of energy, athletes may modify their dietary intake to ensure peak performance both during training and competition.

Strategic Carbohydrate Loading: In endurance sports, loading up on carbs ahead of time optimizes glycogen storage, improving levels of sustained energy.

Protein Intake for Muscle Repair: A vital component of the diet for athletes participating in strength- and power-focused sports, adequate protein intake is essential for both muscle development and repair.

10. Sports-Specific Training for Endurance:

Long-Distance Running Programs: Organized long-distance running or cycling programs help athletes develop the stamina needed for prolonged durations of exercise, such as marathon running and cycling.

Interval Training for High-Intensity Sports: Interval training raises anaerobic thresholds and increases cardiovascular capacity in endurance sports that include short bursts of high-intensity work.

Sports-Specific Terrain Simulations: By simulating the unique terrain and circumstances of a sport, participants may better prepare for the obstacles they would encounter during competition.

11. Technical Expertise Enhancement:
Drills and Repetitions: Consistent drills and repetitions are a key component of sports-specific training, as they help athletes hone their technical abilities and build muscle memory and accuracy in their movement execution.

Video Analysis: Using video analysis to pinpoint areas for technique development enables coaches and athletes to make focused corrections.

Simulated Game Situations: Including simulated game scenarios in team sports training improves team collaboration and decision-making abilities.

12. Adaptability in Training Programs:
Adaptation to the athlete's condition: Training regimens should be flexible to meet individual demands, taking into account the condition and development of each athlete. This is because every athlete is different.

Periodic Reassessment: Making sure training programs are regularly reviewed keeps them in line with an athlete's changing skills, objectives, and any changes to the competitive environment.

Cross-Training to Boost Athletic Output

Coordination across Specialization: The Benefit of Cross-Training

1. Moving Pattern Diversification:
Avoiding Overuse Injuries: By introducing a range of movements, cross-training lowers the risk of overuse injuries brought on by the repeated motions typical of sport-specific training.

Enhanced Range of Motion: Taking part in a variety of activities increases range of motion and general flexibility, which enhances athletic performance and reduces the risk of injury.

Stimulating Neural Adaptation: Diverse movement patterns put the neurological system to the test, which encourages neural adaptation and makes athletes more adaptive and flexible.

2. Developing all-over strength:
Muscle Confusion and Adaptation: By using a variety of muscle groups and movement techniques, cross-training prevents muscles from becoming used to a particular

pattern and encourages the development of general strength.

Balance Between Muscle Groups: Crosstraining helps balance strength and lowers the danger of muscular imbalances by including exercises that focus on underutilized muscle groups.

Decreased Performance Plateaus: By often varying the training stimulus via cross training, performance plateaus are less likely to occur, promoting ongoing development.

3. Prevention of Injury and Rehabilitation:
Active Recovery Techniques: Cross-training is an example of an active recovery strategy that enables athletes to partake in low-impact exercises that increase blood flow and speed up the healing process.

Rehabilitation for Particular Injuries: Crosstraining may help athletes recuperating from particular injuries avoid aggravating the damaged region while keeping their general fitness level high.

Prehabilitation Strategies: By proactively including cross-training in a rehabilitation plan, any vulnerabilities or weaknesses are addressed before they become injuries.

4. Social Rejuvenation and Inspiration:
Reducing Mental Weariness: By offering a mental respite from the unique demands of sport-specific training, cross-

training helps to avoid burnout and reduce mental weariness.

New Challenges and Objectives: Introducing new activities invigorates the athlete's drive and thinking by generating new challenges and objectives.

pleasure and range: Taking part in a range of activities enhances pleasure and variation, which elevates the overall quality of the training experience.

5. Physical Fitness and Aerobic Abilities:
Diverse Cardiovascular Exercises: Cross-training increases aerobic capacity and overall cardiovascular fitness by introducing a diversity of cardiovascular exercises.

Efficient Oxygen Use: Participating in various aerobic exercises enhances oxygen use efficiency, which in turn leads to heightened endurance.

Crossover Benefits: Increased cardiovascular fitness from crosstraining may improve endurance, particularly for a certain activity.

6. Adaptability and skill transfer:
Skill Transfer Across Activities: Developing certain talents in one activity might help you improve your general athleticism and flexibility in other activities.

Enhanced Coordination: Agility and general motor abilities are enhanced via cross-training exercises that test balance and coordination.

Transferable Techniques: An athlete's main sport may benefit from the application or synergy of techniques and movements learned in one discipline.

7. Effective exercise routines:
Integrating high-intensity exercises: Cross-training enables athletes to include time-efficient exercises that provide notable advantages in shorter periods of time, such as high-intensity interval training (HIIT).

Functional Workouts: Cross-training exercises that include functional motions often target many muscle groups at once, increasing the effectiveness of training sessions.

Adaptable to Time Constraints: Time-constrained athletes may modify cross-training programs to meet their schedules, guaranteeing regular exercise.

8. Training load balancing:
times of severe training: Crosstraining provides a means of preserving fitness while lessening the strain on certain joints or muscle groups during times of severe sport-specific training.

Strategic Use in Recovery Weeks: To promote active recovery while preserving physical activity levels, cross-training may be thoughtfully included during recovery weeks.

Cyclical Training Strategy: A cyclical strategy helps balance training loads and avoid overtraining by switching between sport-specific training and cross-training.

9. Building a Team and Variety:
Group Cross-Training Sessions: Including group cross-training sessions improves team dynamics by fostering a feeling of camaraderie among colleagues.

Social Engagement: Cross-training exercises, particularly those carried out in groups, provide chances for social interaction, which improves training enjoyment and strengthens team dynamics.

Team-Building Challenges: Taking part in cross-training activities as a team adds a pleasant competitive aspect that inspires players and strengthens team ties.

10. Strategic Adaptation and Tactical Advantage:
Enhanced Tactical Awareness: Athletes' tactical awareness and decision-making skills are improved via cross-training exercises that mimic the strategic components of several sports.

Adaptability to Varied Conditions: Athletes who are exposed to a variety of training environments are better able to adjust to various surfaces, climates, and unanticipated obstacles they may face during competition.

Strategic Edge Over Specialization: Because cross-trained athletes bring a wider skill set and flexibility to the competition, they may have a strategic edge over athletes who focus only on one sport.

11. Technology Integration for Cross-Training:
Virtual CrossTraining Platforms: Making use of online resources that provide a range of crosstraining exercises, workout guidance, and progress monitoring for a technologically advanced training environment.

Wearable Technology: By integrating wearable technology into cross-training sessions, athletes may improve their workouts by receiving real-time feedback on performance indicators.

CrossTraining Apps: Creation of niche applications with exercise schedules, a range of activities, and tailored training advice for fans of crosstraining.

12. Periodization and Organized Plans for Cross-Training:
Strategic Planning: Including crosstraining in a player's periodized training plan as a whole guarantees a well-rounded strategy that fits with certain performance objectives.

Different Cross-Training Modalities: Putting in place planned programs that include various cross-training modalities to guarantee a thorough approach to physical conditioning.

Input and Adjustments: Regularly evaluating cross-training regimens' efficacy using athlete input and performance indicators and adjusting as needed to ensure ongoing progress.

Difficulties and Things to Think About in CrossFit and Sport-Specific Training:

13. Dangers of Imbalance or Overtraining:
Training Load Monitoring: Constant monitoring of training loads and athlete input guards against overtraining and guarantees well-rounded physical growth.

Periodic Assessments: Frequent evaluations of weak points and imbalances in the muscles enable focused therapies, which lower the risk of overtraining-related ailments.

14. Personalized training schedules:
Customized Approach: Coaches should adapt training schedules to meet the unique requirements and preferences of athletes in order to maximize performance and match personal objectives.

Effective Communication: A collaborative approach to training that takes into account each athlete's preferences and input is ensured by coaches and athletes keeping lines of communication open.

15. Technology Integration:
Tech Literacy: ensuring that coaches and players are techsavvy and know how to use technology properly for tracking, feedback, and training plan improvement.

Data Privacy and Security: Protecting sensitive information gathered by wearable technology and other monitoring devices by putting strong data privacy and security safeguards in place.

16. Synergizing Diversity and Specialization:
Strategic Specialization: giving careful thought to how to combine cross-training with sport-specific training to prevent the emphasis from being lost on critical abilities for competitiveness.

Strategic Cross-Training Periods: Determining certain training cycle points when cross-training might strategically improve overall athleticism without sacrificing talents unique to a given activity.

17. Analytical Framework:
Mental Adjustment: When switching from sport-specific training to cross-training, athletes may need to make mental adaptations that call for psychological assistance and awareness.

Mental Resilience Training: Using mental resilience training to get athletes ready for changes and obstacles brought on by different training philosophies.

Final Thoughts: A Comprehensive Approach to Sports Excellence

Athletes carve out a path of accuracy and variety in the dynamic world of sport-specific and cross-training training, molding themselves into well-rounded contenders. The quest for athletic greatness takes many forms, from developing the specialized abilities needed for a particular activity to accepting the adaptive adaptability fostered by cross-training.

Integrating cross-training with sport-specific training is a smart way to address the mental, physical, and tactical aspects of sports growth. It is evidence of the flexibility and tenacity of athletes who traverse terrain where accuracy and variety collide to realize their greatest potential.

Athletes and coaches must work together to successfully traverse the changing sports and fitness scene, with specialized training and diverse methods playing a critical role. The road to athletic greatness is not a straight line; rather, it is a dynamic dance between the agility required for certain sports and the adaptability developed by cross-training. Through this complex dance, athletes find the perfect balance that helps them reach their highest sporting goals.

Sustaining Long-Term Fitness Achievement: Fostering Adaptive Routines and Sustainable Habits

Starting a Journey towards Lifelong Fitness

Sustaining fitness over the long term is more than just following fad diets and irregular exercise schedules. It's an adventure interwoven with long-lasting routines and dynamic workout program adaptations. This investigation explores the fundamental ideas behind creating long-lasting habits and the skill of modifying workout regimens across a lifetime.

Creating Long-Term Habits

1. Knowing how habits form:
Cue-Routine-Reward Cycle: The basis of habit development is the recognition of the cue that initiates a habit, the routine that follows, and the reward that reinforces the behavior.

Start simple and gradual: Establishing simple, manageable habits and progressively raising their complexity facilitate habit assimilation without overwhelming people.

Regularity in executing an activity fortifies brain connections, causing the habit to become more embedded over time. Consistency is the key.

2. Setting objectives and matching them with values:

Intrinsic Motivation: Fitness objectives that are in line with one's values increase motivation from inside and provide a stronger dedication to long-term success.

SMART Goal Setting: Creating objectives that are specific, measurable, achievable, relevant, and time bound gives ongoing work focus and direction.

Periodic Goal Review: Reviewing goals on a regular basis guarantees their relevance and permits modifications in response to shifting priorities or conditions.

3. Techniques for Mindful Eating:
Intuitive Eating: Adopting an intuitive eating style encourages a sustainable and well-balanced approach to nutrition by paying attention to internal signals of hunger and fullness.

Mindful Meal Planning: Making thoughtful meal plans that take dietary requirements and preferences into account helps people form good eating habits.

Building a Positive Relationship with Food: Promoting a positive and accommodating mindset toward food aids in the development of a long-term, healthy approach to eating.

4. Frequent Exercise as a Way of Life:
Including Daily Movement: Including regular physical exercise in your daily routine, such as riding a bike, walking, or using the stairs, helps you stay fitter overall without the need for regimented training.

Finding Pleasurable Activities: Taking part in activities that make you happy and satisfied increases the chances that you will stick to a regular workout schedule.

Variety in Workouts: Including a range of workouts keeps things interesting and makes being healthy a fun and exciting aspect of daily life.

5. Responsibility and Assistance Frameworks:
Social responsibility: joining exercise groups or sharing fitness objectives with friends fosters a feeling of responsibility that encourages people to stick with their commitment.

Professional counsel: Consulting with health coaches or fitness experts may provide customized counseling and assistance for developing and maintaining healthy behaviors.

Celebrating Milestones: Rewarding yourself for accomplishments along the way to fitness strengthens good habits and motivates you to keep going.

6. Stress Reduction and Emotional Health:
Mind-Body Connection: Understanding how mental and physical health are intertwined highlights how crucial stress management is to general health.

Including Relaxation Techniques: Including techniques like yoga, deep breathing, or meditation improves long-term wellbeing and increases stress resistance.

Adaptive Coping Strategies: Creating adaptive coping mechanisms to handle life's obstacles stops emotional eating or the breakup of good habits when things get tough.

7. Continual Education and Flexibility:
Ongoing Education: Keeping up with changing trends in wellness, nutrition science, and exercise equips people to make wise decisions.

Readjusting Goals: Recognizing that objectives and goals might change over time enables exercise regimens to be readjusted to reflect evolving conditions.

Exploring New Activities: Taking up new wellness or fitness regimens adds diversity, keeps things interesting, and keeps the motivation for leading a healthy lifestyle high.

8. Sleep hygiene and techniques for recovery:
Prioritizing Sleep: Understanding the value of getting enough good sleep to achieve overall fitness and health objectives.

Active Recovery Days: Including days of light exercise or other activities in your schedule promotes muscle recovery and helps you avoid burnout.

Balanced Intensity: Controlling exercise volume and duration while allowing for recovery intervals guards against overtraining and promotes long-term fitness maintenance.

9. Environmental Aspects:

Creating supportive environments: planning living and work areas to encourage healthy practices, including designating a specific spot for exercise or keeping wholesome foods close at hand.

Social and Cultural Pressures: Handling social and cultural pressures by figuring out how to fit one's own routines into the conventions of the community without sacrificing one's own wellbeing.

Sustainability Practices: Using environmentally friendly exercise methods to get about, such as walking or cycling, is in line with both environmental sustainability and individual wellbeing.

10. Contemplation and Adjustment:

Regular self-assessment: Taking stock of routines, accomplishments, and obstacles on a regular basis might reveal areas in need of development and modification.

Flexibility in Approach: Including flexibility in exercise regimens makes it possible to adjust to changes in life and guarantees a long-lasting strategy that can handle a range of situations.

Reassessing Priorities: As life stages change, it's important to reevaluate priorities and modify fitness objectives to ensure that they remain in line with changing circumstances and personal beliefs.

Modifying Exercise Programs over Time

Age-Related Exercise Routines:
Childhood and Adolescence: Promoting an active lifestyle at an early age lays the groundwork for a lifetime of fitness, with a focus on enjoyable and motor skill-enhancing activities.

Adulthood: Adding strength training for bone health, preserving cardiovascular fitness, and modifying exercise regimens to account for shifting responsibilities.

Seniors: tailor exercise routines to concentrate on balance, flexibility, and strength training, recognizing the individual demands and limits associated with age.

Pregnancy and Exercise After Delivery:
Prenatal Workouts: Modifying workout regimens to promote safety and wellbeing while expecting, with an emphasis on activities that enhance general health.

Postpartum Rehabilitation: Restart exercising gradually after giving birth, emphasizing core strengthening, pelvic floor health, and a slow return to prepregnancy fitness levels.

Embracing New Norms: Acknowledging and accepting the physical changes that accompany pregnancy and modifying fitness standards appropriately.

Prevention and Rehabilitation of Injuries:
Rehabilitation Protocols: Adhering to regimented rehabilitation programs after injuries, which include specific exercises and adjustments to avoid recurrence,.

Cross-Training for Injury Prevention: Using a variety of cross-training techniques to lower the chance of overuse injuries brought on by repeated motions.

Listening to the Body: Making adjustments to exercises based on signs of pain or discomfort in order to promote long-term joint and muscle health.

Adjustments to Lifestyle and Career:
Work-Life Balance: Modifying exercise regimens to maintain consistency without unduly stressing out during hectic work seasons or major life transitions.

Including micro exercises: To guarantee continuous physical activity during hectic schedules, look for chances to fit in quick, intensive exercises, or micro workouts.

Adaptability in Method:
Adjusting Training Frequency: Being flexible and aware that there could be times in life when training frequency has to be changed.

Prioritizing Recovery: Giving recovery methods, such as sleep, diet, and relaxation techniques, more priority while under stress or with hectic schedules.

Using Technology to Improve Fitness:
Using Wearable Technology: Adopting wearable fitness trackers or applications to monitor and modify exercises depending on data collected in real time guarantees a customized and flexible strategy.

Virtual Workouts: Including online or virtual exercise platforms gives you versatility in terms of selecting the times and kinds of your workouts, which may accommodate your ever-changing schedule.

Exploring Fitness Apps: To maintain motivation, try out new fitness applications that include a variety of exercises, scalable regimens, and interactive elements.

Changing Up Your Exercise Methods:
Shifting Exercise Focus: Altering between various exercise modalities gradually, e.g., switching from high-impact to low-impact exercises as the body requires them.

Exploring New Fitness Trends: Keeping an open mind to experimenting with new fitness fads or pastimes to keep exercises engaging and flexible enough to accommodate shifting personal tastes.

Combining Modalities: Crafting hybrid exercises that include components from many modalities, offering a comprehensive and balanced approach to physical training.

Participation in social and community activities: Community Workouts: Enrolling in fitness courses or groups in the community may help to create a feeling of camaraderie and shared objectives, which can serve as a source of continuous encouragement.

Taking part in exercise challenges: Taking part in exercise challenges, either by yourself or in a group, promotes consistency and adds a competitive aspect.

Adapting to Social Changes: Modifying exercise regimens to provide ongoing support and involvement throughout the social circle or lifestyle shifts.

Regular fitness evaluations: Regular health checks: conducting fitness evaluations and health checks on a regular basis to detect any changes in health status and modify programs appropriately.

Reevaluating Fitness Goals: Examining how well-aligned existing fitness objectives are with personal values and making necessary adjustments to keep them relevant and motivating.

Tracking Progress: Monitoring progress involves combining objective metrics (like strength increases or endurance improvements) with subjective evaluations (like how one feels both during and after exercise).

Linking Personal Development with Fitness:
Reflecting on Personal Values: Linking exercise regimens with personal development by considering how values are changing and making sure that fitness objectives are in line with larger life goals.

Mind-Body Link: Investigating methods to improve general wellbeing that strengthen the mind-body link, such as mindfulness exercises or holistic wellness strategies.

Adjusting Objectives with Life Phases: Considering that life is dynamic, fitness objectives and regimens should be modified to match various stages, such as professional advancement, family planning, or personal improvement.

Exercises for Cross-Generational Fitness:
Family-Based Activities: Taking part in fitness pursuits that the whole family can enjoy helps to create a culture of health and wellbeing.

Mentorship and guidance: consulting with elder generations who have stayed in good health throughout their lifetimes and applying their knowledge to one's own strategy.

Passing down healthy behaviors: Establishing a legacy of wellbeing within families by modeling and transferring healthy behaviors to subsequent generations.

11. Customizing Dietary Techniques:

Metabolic Changes: Understanding that nutritional requirements and metabolic rates might fluctuate over time and modifying eating patterns accordingly.

Balancing Macronutrients: ensuring an appropriate amount of protein, healthy fats, and carbs while preserving a balance of macronutrients depending on individual requirements.

Nutrient-rich foods: To promote general health, give priority to foods high in nutrients, such as whole grains, lean meats, and a variety of fruits and vegetables.

Integrating Holistic Wellness:

Including Mental Health Practices: Including mental health exercises in exercise regimens, including meditation, to promote overall wellbeing.

Experimenting with Holistic Wellness Modalities: Adding holistic wellness techniques to exercise regimens, such as alternative treatments or practices like aromatherapy or acupuncture,.

Developing a complete wellness plan: Creating a holistic approach to long-term health by creating a complete wellness plan that takes into account mental, emotional, and physical elements.

Difficulties and Things to Take into Account for Maintaining Long-Term Fitness:

Transitions and Difficulties in Life:
Major Life Events: Managing significant life events, such as moving, changing careers, or going through a personal crisis, and modifying exercise regimens to keep them consistent.

Time limits: finding innovative methods to embrace exercise without causing unnecessary stress while balancing time limits throughout hectic life periods.

Mental Health Impact: recognizing how mental health issues affect exercise regimens and getting help when necessary.

Developing muscular abilities:
Aging and Fitness: Understanding that physical abilities may change as one ages and adapting training intensities and regimens to account for these modifications.

Health concerns: adapting workout regimens safely and effectively while managing health concerns; consulting healthcare specialists for advice.

Injury Rehabilitation: Adapting routines during injury rehabilitation, concentrating on activities that aid healing without causing additional damage.

Equilibrium Social Impacts:
Peer Pressure: Keeping personal boundaries, making decisions that are in line with long-term health, and

navigating social situations where unhealthy habits may be common.

Family Dynamics: Striking a balance between individual health objectives, cultural pressures, and family expectations while encouraging candid communication to win support.

External Expectations: Controlling cultural expectations about fitness levels or body appearance means putting one's own wellbeing ahead of outside demands.

Result: An Unwavering Dedication to Health and Well-Being

Sustaining long-term success in fitness is a journey that changes as life changes and is not a destination. It necessitates developing enduring habits, flexibility in exercise regimens, and a dedication to overall wellbeing. The cornerstones of enduring health—listening to the body, living in accordance with one's principles, and accepting change with grace and resilience—remain the same as people move through the many terrains of age, career, family, and personal development.

The quest for long-term fitness achievement becomes a harmonic dance in the symphony of life, where the melody of health blends with the beat of everyday living. It's a dance that flows with the rhythms of life, resonating with the wisdom that true health is a lifetime commitment rather than a temporary accomplishment that enhances each stage of the journey.